LIVABLE LIVES

LIVABLE LIVES

Conversations with the Huntington's Disease Community

Foreword by Jimmy Pollard

CHRISTY DEARIEN

Copyright © 2024 Christy Dearien
All rights reserved. No portion of this book
may be reproduced in any way whatsoever
without the prior written permission of the author.

All storytellers granted the author permission
to share their stories and had multiple opportunities
to review their stories and request edits.

Paperback ISBN: 979-8-9915003-0-2
eBook ISBN: 979-8-9915003-1-9

Cover art: Maggie Dawkins, Instagram @mag.tries.art
Cover design: Natalie Quek, Instagram @studio_nsquek

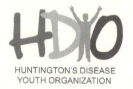

Fifty percent of the author's
net proceeds from the sale of this book
will be donated to HDYO.

www.christydearien.com
Instagram @christydearien

DEDICATED TO

My brother, my parents,
and my grandparents

AND

Continuing the conversation
to improve the lives of
HD families around the world

CONTENTS

Foreword by Jimmy Pollard	1
Author's Note	5
Prologue: A Livable Life	7
Plot Twist: My Story	9
HD 101	34
A Family Disease	50
Children with Huntington's Disease	74
Relating to a Loved One with Huntington's Disease	89
Talking about Huntington's Disease	104
Outlook on Life	126
Genetic Testing	148
Providing Care	175
Research	202
Hope and Meaning	223
Final Reflections	243
Epilogue: A Livable Life	245
Endnotes	247
Acknowledgments	259

FOREWORD

By Jimmy Pollard
HD activist and author of
Hurry Up and Wait!

In the pages ahead, Christy weaves her own story amidst the stories of others from around the world whose lives are touched by Huntington's disease (HD). Within their personal stories there is loss, grief, suffering, and heartbreak. At the same time, there is happiness, gratitude, humor, resilience, and appreciation. Hence, livable lives.

My family is not directly affected by Huntington's disease. However, fate, good luck, education, and a series of wonderful supervisors, employers, and benefactors have given me the unique opportunity for nearly four decades to be fully engaged in the worldwide community of families living with Huntington's. It's been a gift – a humbling gift – to walk beside thousands of individuals who face the challenges HD puts in front of them. Some have HD or have died from their disease. Some are carers. Others I met while working as a professional in nursing homes, assisted living programs, and a state hospital. A few are among my closest, most cherished, and loved friends.

I was honored that Christy asked me to contribute to *Livable Lives*. I have great respect for the work and talent she put into creating this, her labor of love. It's important to tell your story for many reasons. As Christy tells hers, she also creates the opportunity for others to tell theirs. She asked that I try to give a little insight into what I think makes this community so special. I suspect I know this community as well as anyone whose family is not directly touched by HD. It certainly is special. I know it, I sense it, I feel it. I'm immersed in it. But to describe it briefly is daunting.

It's a *community*, obviously and indeed. But as you engage with its members and grow closer to them, the word *community* begins to dissolve as a descriptor from your vocabulary. When you meet someone in the HD community and begin to learn more about them, it's as if you're meeting their family. In fact, it's almost impossible for someone to tell their HD story without telling their family story. When someone is new to HD or makes an initial contact with another person touched by HD, they connect through their family stories. There will be differences, but a bond is created by the common characteristics of their families' stories.

As one meets more members of the *community*, these connections repeat, and one soon realizes that calling it the extended *HD family* better captures the depth of the bond and the essence of their shared experiences than does *community*. Some people reach for the word *tribe*, but tribe, community, or family – they are more than metaphors. The essential bonds of the extended *HD family* are truly worldwide. The shared experiences of living with HD literally transcend borders, cultures, languages, religions, and living conditions.

Families in Venezuela face all the challenges HD brings while living in extreme poverty, and families in Ukraine have organized an HD association while their country is at war. Families in other countries live with social stigma for having a genetic disease, and many reach out for help in teaching their towns and villages that HD is not contagious. Despite such profound differences, shared experience connects them all – one worldwide extended family.

You'll often hear this community or family described as *resilient*. If I had to pick a single descriptor, yes, perhaps it's resilient. But there's much more to these individuals and families than the characteristic of getting back up every time they're knocked down. Remember, it takes a lot of being knocked down and getting back up before people even realize that you are resilient! That resilience entails persevering through all kinds of challenges for a very long time.

In these pages, you'll read examples of resilience in Christy's story and those of the people with whom she spoke. There are countless other stories, though, that you won't read about here or elsewhere. They belong to people who are well along on their HD roads and no longer able to articulate their stories due to the challenges they face in HD's later years. When I worked in nursing homes, these individuals were the first to welcome me to the extended HD family and introduce me to their own families, despite their impaired speech, physical infirmities, and cognitive challenges.

Their stories are untold, but they persevere despite all the difficulties that HD puts in front of them, moment-to-moment, day in and day out, for years. With a stamina that opened my eyes, they persevere. Dependent on others, but still a most livable life for these resilient souls, even in the later years of their HD roads. It's the same resilience woven through the stories in *Livable Lives*.

Walking one's long HD road, or walking alongside one you love, is often a lonely experience. While we are blessed with access to world-class medical and psychiatric care and the support of allied health professionals and rehabilitation therapists, much of Huntington's disease still happens in the home. Perhaps you're helping your spouse on the toilet, or your loved one is irritable, has a short fuse, and is yelling at you, again, as you try to help them. Perhaps you're quietly reflecting on why something you've done quickly a thousand times now seems so complicated. Perhaps you're wondering why you can't summon the energy to simply begin your day, run an errand, or make a phone call.

These are lonely experiences that over time – sometimes years, sometimes across generations – become profoundly lonesome experiences. Yet, individuals and families endure them. Instead of talking about loneliness, though, HD families persevere by getting to work, managing their homes and kids, worrying about finances, and navigating healthcare systems, all in the face of so many lonely moments. This is resilience, too, but with an unseen depth that we may not usually associate with the word. Through their collective resilience, pooled all over the world, they have found each other and founded HD associations, raised the money to keep them going for decades, and fully partnered with physicians and scientists in HD-related research. It is something to appreciate.

That's my humble observation of what makes this a special group, community, extended family, or tribe. I don't pretend to understand how or why, but this family is welcoming to a degree that I've never encountered elsewhere. Having seen it all, having weathered storm after storm over their lives and across generations, they don't judge others. They simply know that anyone facing an HD road is doing their best. No judgment. Only warm welcoming embraces.

You will hear my professional colleagues and I talk about how much we've learned from this resilience, perseverance, and endurance in HD families. There is so much we apply to our own private lives. This is not lip service. Take us at our word! Walking alongside HD families, we've seen the challenges HD creates in every dimension of families' lives. We've seen that all lives are livable and can be lived with happiness, joy, and wonder. Simply read on...

– Jimmy Pollard

AUTHOR'S NOTE

L*ivable Lives* is the book I wish I had when I first learned about Huntington's disease (HD). I remember looking for a single source that not only described the disease but could also help me understand the complicated and overwhelming issues my family was facing.

- If you recently discovered that you or a loved one is impacted by Huntington's disease, I hope the stories in *Livable Lives* help you understand that you are not alone.
- If you are impacted by Huntington's disease but have not yet engaged with others from the HD community, I encourage you to find opportunities to join this special community. I have no doubt that you will be welcome.
- If you have been part of the HD community for a long time, I hope you see your own experiences reflected in *Livable Lives* and are reminded of just how important it is to connect with and support each other.
- If you find it hard to describe Huntington's disease and all it entails, I hope this book provides a starting point for conversations with family members, friends, doctors, therapists, teachers, social workers, and others. It is important that the people around us

understand the complicated nature of this disease, so we don't have to feel isolated and alone.
- And if you are reading *Livable Lives* to learn about Huntington's disease, I hope this book answers your questions.

Please be aware that *Livable Lives* touches on many challenging topics. They include, but are not limited to, verbal or physical abuse, suicide, mental illness, genetic testing, caregiving, decisions related to having children, and complicated relationships. **If you are having a difficult time or need support, please seek help** from a family member, a friend, a therapist, or an HD organization. Resources for connecting with HD organizations are available throughout this book, but a good place to start is the Huntington's Disease Youth Organization (hdyo.org).

The information presented in *Livable Lives* **is not a substitute for medical advice,** so please consult your doctor about any health concerns.

Finally, to maintain privacy, some *Livable Lives* storytellers have chosen to use pseudonyms or first names only in their stories.

With that, welcome to the HD community!

PROLOGUE: A LIVABLE LIFE

Liv-a-ble life [ˈli-və-b(ə)l lif] *noun*

1. The period when a gene-positive or at-risk person can live the life they want to live before Huntington's disease (HD) symptoms appear.
2. A life lived with intention and meaning in response to an uncertain or daunting future.
3. A high quality of life for loved ones who have Huntington's disease.

In the last several years, I've had many conversations with members of the HD community to learn as much as I could about how Huntington's disease impacts individuals and families. The term, *livable life*, came to my attention in a conversation with a young woman who knows she has the expanded gene that causes Huntington's disease. She talked about having a short amount of time to live the life she wants to live before HD symptoms appear sometime in middle age. She calls this period her *livable life*.

In some ways, knowing she carries the expanded gene – knowing she is gene positive – limits her plans, especially her career aspirations. A PhD program is off the table because she wants to start her career soon and have time to save for future medical costs. In other ways, it adds value to her life because she knows she needs to make things happen now. She makes intentional decisions to live a full and meaningful life today – a *livable life* of her choice.

The term, *livable life*, captures a lot of what I heard in my conversations as people talked about how they approach their lives, whether they're at risk for Huntington's disease, gene positive, gene negative, or have family members with the disease. A *livable life* might mean making plans to prepare for the challenges that lie ahead. It might mean focusing on the present because it is too hard to think about the past or the future, or it might mean doing things that bring joy to loved ones who have Huntington's disease. On the most difficult days, a *livable life* might mean doing whatever it takes to get through the day, or even the next hour.

Above all, a *livable life* encompasses the many ways those in the HD community cope with a life that includes this devastating disease. As you get to know the people who shared their stories with me, you will come to understand just how important it is to members of the HD community to create and maintain their own *livable life*.

PLOT TWIST: MY STORY

When my older brother was diagnosed with Huntington's disease at age 49, my family's story changed in an instant. We had hoped that finding an explanation for my brother's symptoms would help him get better, but that hope was crushed when we learned he had a terminal neurological disease. Not only that, but Huntington's disease is genetic, so we also learned that many people in my family – including me and my kids – might carry the genetic mutation that causes the disease. My brother's diagnosis was just the beginning of a journey to understand my family's past, present, and future with this disease and the losses that come with it.

I had never heard of Huntington's disease, so I scoured the internet and got a crash course on what we were facing. Certain things stood out. It is a fatal disease that devastates families, not just individuals. Every child of someone with Huntington's disease has a 50-50 chance of inheriting it. Huntington's disease is neurodegenerative and has a long list of potential physical, cognitive, and behavioral symptoms. Chorea, which means *dance* in Latin, is a hallmark symptom of Huntington's disease that is characterized by involuntary movements of the face, limbs, and torso. Symptoms typically start in middle age but may start in childhood or old age. There is currently no cure.

For many family diseases, genetics are one part of an equation that includes environmental, social, and other causal factors. Many people know they have a predisposition to cancer or heart disease, for example, but their chance of developing those diseases is not set in stone. They can exercise, eat well, and get regular checkups to reduce their risk and give themselves the best chance of living a healthy life. However, genetics are the *only* factor that determines if someone will develop Huntington's disease. Those who inherit an expanded HD gene will develop the disease unless they die of another cause before symptoms begin. Those who inherit a normal HD gene will not develop the disease. It's non-negotiable.

My new reality

When I was new to the HD world, I wondered how my brother's diagnosis could have come as a surprise. Most people know when a disease runs in their family, and it seems this would be especially true for Huntington's disease because it does not skip generations. However, my family is not alone in unexpectedly discovering we are an HD family. In my conversations with the HD community, I talked with many people who grew up knowing nothing about Huntington's disease because a family member with the disease was adopted or misdiagnosed, or their family didn't talk openly about it.

In my family, we now know that my grandpa was misdiagnosed with Parkinson's disease, and my dad's HD symptoms were never properly understood or diagnosed before he died of cancer. My brother's diagnosis was the first time we had a name for this disease that has impacted my family for generations. As I learned more about Huntington's disease, my anxiety about what the future held for my family grew. Due to the hereditary nature of the disease, 10 members of my family could potentially carry the expanded gene that causes

Huntington's disease, including me, both of my brothers, and each of our kids. What if all of us carried the expanded gene?

Once I was over the initial shock of learning I was at risk for Huntington's disease, I didn't share the news widely. This was partly because I'm a private person, but also because letting people know I was at risk often meant answering questions I wasn't ready to answer. When I did share, some people offered words of encouragement, others were at a loss as to what to say, and then there were a few who were comfortable sharing their thoughts about what I should do. I could know my gene status through a simple blood test at any time, so they would tell me I should get tested right away. At the very least, they knew they wouldn't hesitate to do so. They were confident about this. Wouldn't it be better to know what I was dealing with so I could make plans? If I knew I was gene positive, I could get my finances in order and make sure I did things I wanted to while I could. Why wait?

Before I learned I was at risk, this way of thinking about my future would have made sense to me because I'm a planner. I soon found out, however, that being able to take a genetic test to know your future is no blessing and presents a dilemma for those who are at risk for Huntington's disease. Without testing, there's no way to know if you will have a long life that looks normal, or a life cut short by a disease that takes away so much. With testing, you receive either relief or crushing news. With or without testing, there's no way to know when symptoms might appear or what the collection of symptoms might look like. I advise those who don't have to make this decision to drop the notion that you know what you would do. When given the chance, it is daunting to peek into the future to know what is coming.

Deciding whether to pursue genetic testing is far from straightforward for those of us who have to face this decision head on. When it was my turn, I had several reasons for not testing right away. I honestly didn't know if I could cope with a positive result. Early on, I met a young woman who was gene positive but presymptomatic. Her sadness was palpable and heavy. I wondered how she faced each day knowing what was coming. I didn't think I could bear the truth if I tested positive, and I knew I could plan for my future without getting tested. I could make smart financial decisions and plan my days and years to get the most out of life, which is what we should all do anyway. I didn't need to know my gene status to live each day as if it mattered. Without testing, I didn't have to carry the burden of my worst-case scenario.

It was also difficult to contemplate what a positive test result would mean for my family. I had a fear of facing Huntington's disease alone if caring for me became too much for my husband and kids, but that was countered by the fear of making them go down that path with me. For the first few years, not knowing was easier than knowing the worst.

During those early months after my brother's diagnosis, I felt the presence of an alternate version of myself – a new version that was at risk for Huntington's disease. I didn't want to interact with this new version of myself, and yet I couldn't get away from her. She was always there, like an unwelcome guest, waiting for me to notice. I could push my thoughts about Huntington's disease and genetic testing aside for periods of time, but they always returned.

Gradually, after many months, being at risk for Huntington's disease became a part of me, a new me. While the old me could think about growing old or planning for adventures, the new me didn't know what to plan for. Were symptoms just around the corner or maybe even already present? Was I on the precipice of a long and slow decline? Was my future one where I could choose my path, or was it one where my ability to do so would be whittled away little by little? And the question that was hardest to face: had I passed the same fate along to my two boys? Their future was bound to mine, and that thought was too much to bear.

A link to the past

I have few memories of my grandpa because I never got the chance to know him. I didn't even meet my grandparents until I was seven years old when our family drove from Idaho to Connecticut to visit them. My grandpa was living in a psychiatric hospital at the time, and I didn't understand why he was there. It was unnerving as a seven-year-old to walk down the hallway of his ward and wonder what was happening behind all those solid closed doors with tiny windows.

I don't know if my recollection of something that happened when I was seven is accurate, and I don't know if my interpretation of what my grandpa was thinking is anywhere close to the truth. In my memory, though, it seemed like my grandpa knew he was meeting me and my younger brother for the first time even though he was no longer able to speak to let us know that. My grandpa sat quietly in his wheelchair and stared at us intently while my family carried on a conversation, but when it was time for him to go back to his room, he screamed as he was wheeled away.

That was my only interaction with my grandpa until my grandparents moved to my hometown a couple of years later. My grandpa moved into a local nursing home, and I visited him periodically with my family. We took him ice cream and strawberries from our garden to eat on the patio, and again, he sat quietly while we talked. My grandpa passed away about six months later at the age of 79. Given his collection of physical and psychiatric symptoms and the hereditary nature of Huntington's disease, we now know my grandpa's Parkinson's diagnosis was a misdiagnosis.

My memories of my grandpa are limited to a handful of visits in which we couldn't interact in a way that allowed us to develop any sort of bond or relationship. I never had a conversation with my grandpa. He never gave me a hug, and I never sat on his lap to read a story together. I've come to understand that *not knowing* a loved one is a central facet of

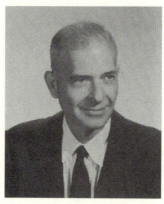
My grandpa.

Huntington's disease. Instead of leaving my knowledge of my grandpa to a few vague childhood recollections, I wanted to know him better. I sought out whatever was available to round out this person who should have been a central part of my upbringing. I read my aunt's family history account and asked family members what my grandpa was like before he developed Huntington's disease.

Learning about my grandpa in this way won't make up for truly knowing him as a person, but I've discovered details that help me imagine what he was like. I now know that my grandpa was reserved and patient. He had a wry smile and a great sense of humor. My grandpa loved music and played the trumpet in the Yale band; he also knew how to play the accordion. He enjoyed building and fixing things, and he rigged up a system to play music throughout the house. My grandpa was smart and ran his own business. He once made a hole-in-one in a round of golf. I also learned that he tried to commit suicide at least once when he still lived in Connecticut. These are small things to know, but they're all I have.

If only we had known

My dad overcame a lot as a kid. He contracted polio at a football game when he was in the fourth grade, just a few years before a vaccine was available. He didn't get sick enough to need an iron lung, but he did lose some mobility. He eventually regained the function of everything except his dominant right arm. My dad had to relearn how to do everything with only his left arm: big tasks like eating, dressing, and writing, and small tasks like opening lids and carrying things one-handed. In my mind, he could do anything anyone else could, but apparently, changing diapers one-handed was a challenge. He loved to fish, ski, and explore the outdoors. He smiled a lot – enough that my high school friend said he reminded her of an elf.

One of my favorite early memories of my dad involved eating popsicles together on our front steps on a hot summer evening and watching the sunset while the heat of the sun still emanated from the concrete. My little brother and I doggie-piled my dad on the grass and wrestled with him to our delight. Another favorite was when he would come upstairs from the basement wearing a mummy mask to scare us. These carefree memories exist outside of the complicated feelings I had about my dad once Huntington's disease took hold. I don't know when Huntington's disease changed my dad from the person I knew when I was very young to the person I knew as a teenager and young adult. He changed gradually at first and had more dramatic changes as his disease progressed.

When my dad died of cancer at age 57, he was in what I now recognize as the middle stage of Huntington's disease. He had been having HD symptoms for about a decade. He had classic physical, cognitive, and behavioral symptoms of Huntington's disease, but without a known family history, his doctors looked elsewhere when making their diagnoses. Now that I know what chorea looks like, there's no doubt my dad had these distinctive involuntary movements. They stand out in my memory even though he died when I was a young adult. My dad would twist his torso in a way that included a strange lift of his shoulder, and he seemed to constantly move his feet and adjust his position when sitting in his recliner. His doctor attributed his physical symptoms to post-polio syndrome, which includes muscle atrophy, progressive weakness, and fatigue, but the doctor never mentioned my dad's strange movements.

Thinking back, I know my dad had at least some cognitive decline. He became less engaged in conversations, and he sometimes had an absent stare that I now see in my older brother from time to time. Work became more and more challenging, and he started having difficulty interacting with colleagues. He was sent home from a work trip once, though it was never clear to my mom what happened. He had always been a model employee, so none of this made sense. My dad was let go from his job when I was a junior in college.

My dad's behavioral symptoms had a big impact on his relationship with my mom, my siblings, and me. Small things, like if I spilled some juice, could set off a huge reaction. I remember two incidents when I was in elementary school, when his reaction to whatever I did scared me – something that was out of character for him. At times, my dad seemed completely unreasonable and unwilling to budge. Without giving any reason, we were told we couldn't go out with friends or have them over. My younger brother wasn't allowed to travel with my dad to our uncle's funeral. As my dad's HD symptoms progressed and his way of thinking became more rigid, I hit my teenage years and there were plenty of arguments even though I was an agreeable teenager.

My dad also developed an assortment of odd behaviors. He compulsively checked door locks and let the dog in and out of the back yard over and over throughout the day – something I know the dog appreciated. He would set a timer and walk around inside the house until it went off instead of going out into the neighborhood for a walk. I remember finding my dad in the kitchen with all four stove burners turned on red hot, just watching them. I also remember my grandma coming in the front door to find my dad standing on top of one of the end tables in the living room. She immediately told him to get down. None of these behaviors were dangerous or threatening, but they weren't normal.

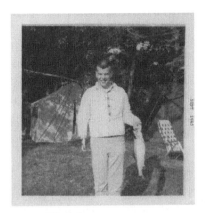

My dad as a young man.

One month after my high school graduation, my dad had his first major break from reality just days after his mom died. He started hallucinating, so we took him to the emergency room. This was the beginning of many years of working with a psychiatrist who never figured out that my dad's psychiatric symptoms were caused by a neurodegenerative disease. My dad's symptoms didn't match any disorder outlined by the American Psychiatric Association. His psychiatrist considered schizophrenia as a diagnosis, but eventually settled on psychotic depression as the closest fit. My mom could never figure out why no one seemed to know exactly what was wrong with my dad. I don't know why the psychiatrist didn't observe my dad's chorea and realize something else was going on. I can't help but think he should have noticed movements I still remember decades later.

My dad's second major break from reality happened the summer after I graduated from college. A few days before we were supposed to leave for my older brother's wedding, my dad physically cornered my mom in their bedroom and wouldn't let her leave. My mom went to the hospital with chest pain later that day and was kept for observation. When I woke that night to the sound of my dad mumbling outside my door, I got up to see how he was doing. I sat at the top of the stairs for a long time, while he stood in the hallway repeating over and over that the house was falling down and he didn't know what to do. All I could do was reassure him that everything was okay, which did little to appease his anxiety or convince him that the house was fine. By this time, my dad acting strangely wasn't new to me, so I wasn't afraid. I was just concerned for his wellbeing and felt unable and unequipped to help him.

The next day was possibly the most difficult day of my life. When my mom was released from the hospital, she and I went to my maternal grandma's house. After several conversations between my mom and my parents' doctor about my dad's uncharacteristically aggressive behavior, the doctor asked a judge to issue an order to involuntarily commit my dad to the behavioral health center. That afternoon, my dad called my mom to say the police were at the door and he didn't know what to do. My mom had to tell him to go with them. That was a hard phone call to listen to – I knew it was difficult for them both. Our neighbor and good friend later told my mom he cried when he saw the police bring my dad out to the police car in handcuffs. I'm sure my dad was scared and confused by what was happening.

I took my dad's suitcase to the behavioral health center later that day, and I was asked to sign papers to admit him. I don't remember anything about the person who sat with me to go through this process. I don't even remember if they were male or female. I mostly remember how I felt: confused, conflicted, heartbroken. I was 21 years old. I didn't feel old enough to sign paperwork to commit my dad to a psychiatric unit without his consent, and yet there I was. I went through the motions because I didn't know what else to do. I signed papers, and I watched this person go through my dad's suitcase to remove items that could be used to harm himself or others, including a razor, a belt, and shoelaces.

While I went through this process, my dad was in an adjoining room, and we could see each other through a small window in a door that separated us. He peered through the glass with a pleading look in his eyes as he repeated my name over and over. I felt like I had betrayed him. Thirty years later, these small details are clear as day in my memory.

We left town the next day without my dad to go to my brother's wedding, and my dad spent the next month in the behavioral health center.

My dad was diagnosed with cancer three years later. In the months after this diagnosis, he seemed more like his old self. I'm not sure why. At the time, I thought the harsh reality of cancer must be what helped ground him. No matter the reason, this time was a gift. I cherish the last few months we had with him. I was able to return home to visit my dad every month, and we went on day trips to places we had visited many times during my childhood, like Craters of the Moon, Mesa Falls, and Big Springs.

I'm grateful that some of my last memories with my dad are in places he loved and that brought back happy memories from my childhood. It had been a long time since I had enjoyed spending time with him. I took my last photograph of my dad on one of those trips. This was before the days of digital photography, so I had to wait to get the film processed. A few weeks after my dad died, I picked up the processed photos. There, in the middle of the bunch, was my dad, looking right at me one last time. I treasure that photo to this day. It's in a small frame on a bookshelf, right next to pictures of my kids and my mom. I walk by it often and notice his smile.

My dad has been gone for more than half my lifetime and practically all my adult life. I often wonder how different our lives would have been

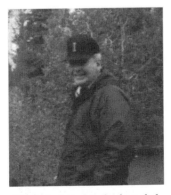

The last photo I took of my dad.

if we had known we were an HD family. So many things about my dad and grandpa made a lot of sense once we knew where their psychiatric and other symptoms originated. If I'd had this understanding when my dad was alive, I can't help but think I would have been more sympathetic to how difficult things were for him. His changing personality and progressing symptoms were beyond his control and not his fault.

I used to think my dad was unlucky to have had polio as a kid and then die so young of cancer. Now that we know he had Huntington's disease, cancer seems like a blessing in disguise because my dad didn't have to experience the final and most difficult stage of Huntington's disease. It would be 18 years, however, before we would understand that we are an HD family.

Now we know

When my dad started having pronounced mental health issues, I worried that his psychiatric symptoms and my grandpa's stay in a psychiatric hospital were somehow related, but my dad and grandpa never received diagnoses that explained what they had in common. I didn't know they shared a genetic disease, and yet I had a feeling – an ominous feeling – that what had happened to them could also happen to me and my siblings. I had no idea just how prophetic this feeling was until my older brother started having similar symptoms.

My brother has a warm personality and a great sense of humor. One of his childhood friends described him as, "one of the smartest, funniest, and most caring people I've met who was always able to crack people up with some of the most oddball but spot-on funny lines I've ever heard." My brother is six years older than me, so my childhood memories center around him being the big brother who was often hanging out with friends. He played a lot of soccer and baseball. He did cool things like making an ice rink in the backyard, building a massive snow fort next to the driveway, and setting up a carnival in the yard for the neighborhood kids. As a young adult, he caught the travel bug and took several extended trips abroad. When I realized my brother was unlikely to ever travel again, I placed a note from him in my suitcase. There's nothing special about the note itself, but keeping it tucked in my suitcase feels like I'm taking him with me on my travels.

Like my dad, my brother's symptoms started gradually and included uncharacteristic reactions to situations, increasingly rigid ways of thinking and relating to others, increased anxiety and depression, and unusual movements. He told my mom he was having trouble focusing on his work, something that reminded her of conversations she had with my dad years ago. My brother's driving was possibly the earliest sign that something was wrong. Several years before his diagnosis, he started to jerk the steering wheel and hit the gas and brake pedals repeatedly. This made for a very bumpy ride. As symptoms crept in, he sought answers from a variety of doctors, but it was at least four years before a neurologist looked at all the pieces and put them together.

Many people with Huntington's disease don't notice some of their own symptoms, and my brother was no exception. Several months before his diagnosis, I arrived at his home the same afternoon he had an MRI that had been ordered by the neurologist who would later diagnose

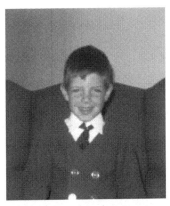

My brother as a child.

his Huntington's disease. By this time, my brother's movements were hard to ignore. He was cheerful when he arrived back at his house, and he chuckled as he told us the MRI technician had asked if he'd be able to stay still for the duration of the scan. To him, it was a funny question because of course he could. In my mind, however, it was obvious that sitting still for any length of time was impossible for him.

My brother's symptoms continued to progress after his diagnosis, and by Christmas-time a couple of years later, leaving home caused him so much anxiety that he almost didn't make it out of the house to travel to our mom's house for the holiday. During this visit, he and I had one of our last connected conversations. He wanted to know how I was doing. Even though he was the one facing Huntington's disease head on, he genuinely cared about how I was coping with being at risk. He was being a good big brother, just as he always had been. My brother's condition went downhill quickly after that trip.

Perseveration is a common symptom of Huntington's disease that is often described as getting stuck on ways of thinking or doing things. After that Christmas visit, my brother became so fixated on pain in his hands and feet that it became debilitating. His pain limited him to walking short distances – maybe a block or two – before he had to sit down. On a trip to Vancouver Island, my mom and I waited patiently whenever he stopped, set up his folding chair on the sidewalk, and rested a while before we moved on. He eventually started using a wheelchair to get around his house, and it wasn't long before he stopped walking except to move between his wheelchair and his bed or the car, for example.

My brother soon developed an intense suicidal ideation, but he was unable to gather his thoughts together well enough to figure out how to do it. One day, he called me and quickly said, "I'm going to kill myself... I love you... Goodbye." Click... I didn't have a chance to say anything before he hung up. Several family members received the same phone call. I knew he had perseverated on suicide for quite a while, so his phone call wasn't a surprise. Even though I knew he wasn't cognitively capable of killing himself, hearing those words was heart-wrenching. My brother's phone calls were an indication of how severe his depression had become. I phoned my sister-in-law immediately to be sure she knew about the call. We all felt incapable of helping him in a meaningful way.

Soon after, with no end in sight to his deep depression and suicidal ideation, my brother spent one month in a psychiatric ward before moving to a group home. With appropriate medication prescribed by a doctor with knowledge of Huntington's disease, his psychiatric symptoms improved, and he settled into a new normal. Any change in routine or surroundings was hard for him, so the group home became the place where he felt most comfortable. For the next several years, he rarely left other than to return home for a few hours on Thanksgiving or Christmas, and he didn't always make it home even then.

My brother's symptoms seem to cycle between periods of swift decline that can last a couple of months and longer periods where his symptoms seem to plateau. During periods of rapid decline, his sleep patterns are disrupted, he spends more time in his room, and he becomes less engaged. His depression deepens, and he sometimes has suicidal ideation. When I visit him during these periods, he speaks very little and seems so far away. Sometimes my brother's changing symptoms can be addressed by a change in medication, but twice these rapid changes have resulted in extended stays in a psychiatric ward. The periods of decline are alarming, and each time we wonder how different he will be when the decline levels out. During these periods, it is hard to ignore what the disease is taking away from him and our family. During the plateaus, however, it is easy to fall into a new rhythm and simply focus on spending time together.

My brother has changed considerably since his diagnosis 10 years ago. He now relies on others to prepare his meals and help him shower, dress, and use the bathroom. He is no longer able to write, use a cell phone, or venture out into the world on his own. It's not easy to understand my brother's speech, and he typically only responds to questions or prompts from others – usually with very short answers. I can't remember the last time I heard a spontaneous sentence from him that wasn't an answer to someone's question. His chorea is noticeable but managed relatively well by medication. The muscles that help my brother swallow are getting weaker, which increases his risk of choking.

I live 300 miles from my brother, but I try to visit every couple of months. I know I need to focus on our time together and not take it for granted. When my brother could still text on his phone, he sent me messages like, "Yes!" and "Amdojbf good" and "I did +@." In August 2021, I received my last text from him. It was simple: "Thanks @." I miss my brother's enthusiastic text messages with excessive use of symbols and exclamation points, and I know this is just one of the many lasts we'll experience.

When my kids were little, I wondered when I would pick them up and carry them for the last time or when they would crawl into my lap to read one last story together. I knew those things would happen less frequently over time, and one day – without my knowledge – they would happen for the last time. This transition would be sad, but it would mean they were growing up and becoming independent. Now, I wonder when I'll have my last verbal response from my brother. I imagine it will be much like my kids getting older. It will change gradually over time, become less frequent, and then one day – without my realizing it – it will be the last time.

Despite my brother's decline, I've been surprised that there have been some positive changes as well. After recent medication changes, moving to a new group home, and possibly a change in the part of his brain that made him perseverate, he seems happier and more relaxed. He's now willing to go out and experience the world. His family takes him to restaurants, movies, and concerts, and they've even gone to see his favorite sports teams play. I don't always understand the changes I see in my brother. I know Huntington's disease is degenerative, so anything that is lost cannot be regained. It's easy to assume the changes we see are directly tied to his brain slowly dying, but then something will happen that seems like a small miracle.

I was surprised recently when my brother told his caregiver he wanted to talk to me. When I called, I couldn't believe the conversation we had. He answered my questions quickly and sometimes with complete sentences. When I asked what he had been up to, he responded, "The Mariners made it to the playoffs." I quickly counted in my head. Seven words! It had been years since I'd heard seven words in a row. Another response about a women's FIFA World Cup game we went to years ago was, "They scored a lot of goals." My mind was racing as I tried to remember what he was saying while still thinking of things to tell him or ask about. We talked for about five minutes, and most of his responses were his usual ones like, "I do," and "Oh yeah." I was elated he had reached out to me and shocked that I got to experience this rare conversation.

I wonder how my brother experiences the world. I wonder what is happening in his brain that he is unable to express outwardly, and what happens to allow small breakthrough miracles like our recent phone conversation. Does he have an ongoing conversation in his head, or has Huntington's disease dampened his internal voice as well? I hope he has a rich inner world he can explore. Over the years, it has become gradually more difficult to recognize my brother behind his HD symptoms as he engages less in conversation. He doesn't express much through facial expressions now, except when we first walk into his room to greet him, or when we trigger a memory or say something he finds funny. At these moments, though, his face lights up or he laughs. These moments make me happy, but I know that they, too, will come to an end one day.

Looking to my future

More than four years passed between learning I was at risk for Huntington's disease and deciding to get tested – four years in which I thought about the pros and cons of genetic testing every single day. I knew I'd likely get tested one day, either to confirm a diagnosis or when I was old enough that I was somewhat confident I'd escaped the disease.

In the end, my decision centered around wanting to give my two boys a chance to know they were okay as they entered young adulthood – that their futures were theirs to navigate however they wanted. Up until this point, I felt like my absence of symptoms served as a buffer for them – if I was okay, they were okay – but that was no longer enough. I wanted to let them off the hook if I could.

Before initiating the genetic testing process, I wanted my kids' permission because my test result had a direct impact on them. If I received a negative result, all three of us would know we were gene negative. If I received a positive result, however, we would know that I would develop Huntington's disease, and my kids would continue to be at risk with a 50-50 chance that they had inherited the disease. If either of my kids had said they didn't want to know, I would have abandoned the process and remained at risk, but they both supported my decision to go ahead.

When I first told my husband I was thinking of getting tested, he gave me his full support. After witnessing my brother's changes over many years, my husband didn't see any of the same changes in me. He was certain my test result was going to be negative. This was enough to allay his fears but not mine. I had to talk my husband into imagining what our lives would be like if we learned I was going to develop Huntington's disease. Knowing my gene status would affect my outlook, my relationships, and how I made decisions. It would set the course for the rest of our lives, and there would be no going back, no way of unknowing. I needed us both to be equally prepared for either possibility.

If I received a positive test result, I knew I would need time to absorb that knowledge before sharing my news with anyone else, so my husband and kids were the only ones who knew I was getting tested. It took me several weeks to get up the nerve to schedule an appointment. When my husband and I first met with the genetic counselor, he confirmed that HD symptoms can appear at an earlier age in each successive generation, especially when the parent with Huntington's disease is male. At the time I tested, I was about the same age my dad was when he started exhibiting HD symptoms, and I was several years older than my brother had been. However, there was no guarantee I was in the clear.

When my husband and I met with the genetic counselor several weeks later to get my test result, I thought I knew what to expect. I had done my research. In my imagined scenario, the counselor would have a sealed envelope containing my test result and, like me, he would have no idea what my result would be. Up until the moment the envelope was opened, I would have the option of backing out. The counselor's expression would give nothing away and wouldn't sway my decision because he wouldn't know if I was gene positive or gene negative. I thought no one would know the result until I was ready.

As we walked into the genetic counselor's office, the counselor verified that I was certain I wanted to know my result. I did. I'd taken my time making this decision, and I didn't want to go through the stress of waiting for a test result again. My affirmative response was followed immediately by the genetic counselor saying, "Well, I can tell you that your test result is good. You don't have the expanded gene. Neither you nor your children can get Huntington's disease."

That was it. It took less than a minute. There was no dramatic opening of a sealed envelope. There were no harrowing moments of waiting for papers to be pulled from the envelope and scanned to find my result. I don't think I'd even settled into my seat before he finished talking. The counselor had known my result before I walked into his office. Even though I'd imagined this moment many times, I was stunned. There was nothing wrong with how I received my test result, and it had no bearing on how I felt about my experience. It just wasn't what I expected. All I could think to say in return was, "Thank you."

Immediately after receiving my negative result, I thought I was supposed to feel relief, but I mostly felt numb. Before getting tested, I had considered in detail the specific moment when I would receive my test result. I had focused my attention on how I would cope with a positive result and what my life would be like if I developed Huntington's disease. I knew I needed to be prepared for that outcome. I hadn't given much thought to how I would respond to a negative result.

Testing negative was supposed to mean that I was going to be okay, so I didn't realize it would come with its own challenges. Even now, I'm not sure how I could have prepared for the complex emotions that came with learning I had a chance to have a healthy future.

Receiving what might seem like the best news of my life was emotional. I cried for days. The testing process and its aftermath are both intense. The best way I can explain it to others is that belonging to an HD family is like being on a sinking ship. The ship is going down slowly, and there's no avoiding the worst-case scenario in the end. Testing negative for Huntington's disease meant that my kids and I suddenly found safe and secure seats in the lifeboat. While we were safe, there was nothing we could do to change the course for the people we love who are still on that sinking ship. For now, there is no lifeboat for them. We continue to watch that ship sink slowly with them on board, and there's no happiness in that.

Telling people my good news was much more emotional than I'd expected. It was easy to tell my mom because I knew she had carried the burden of worrying about me and my boys. My news meant that three more of us were safe. It was difficult to tell my older brother and his family. I knew it would bring up a lot of emotions for them because I was, in a sense, leaving them behind. They were happy for me and my kids, but I worried they might feel more alone in facing Huntington's disease. Telling my friends was also difficult. As they told me they were thrilled to hear my good news, I found that happiness was not what I felt. I was grateful for my negative result, and I was relieved my kids were okay, but happiness was not the right emotion, and there was no celebration.

While my husband never thought I was gene positive, he confessed that my negative test result eased thoughts he had tucked away over the years. He remembers asking himself, "Did that piece of doubt in the back of my head just disappear?" He knew there was a possibility I was gene positive, but he hadn't dwelled on it. He had been comfortable assuming I was okay, so he had looked to the future as if that was the case. His theory has always been that there's nothing to worry about until there's

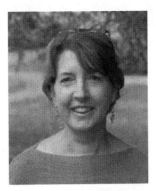
And this is me.

something to worry about. Never mind that we had different ideas about what was worthy of worry. While being at risk worried me, he wasn't going to worry unless I had symptoms or tested positive. If I had gotten a positive result, he said, "It would have changed everything. We were given the straight road – you don't get to choose which one you take." The outcome of my genetic test was always out of our hands.

After testing negative, it took at least a year for my anxiety and fear of potentially having Huntington's disease to ease. Being at risk had become such an integral part of my identity and had occupied so much of my emotional energy, that it took time to let it go. Finally, the possibility of having Huntington's disease is no longer a constant just-below-the-surface worry. I no longer have to consider a future in which my kids and I will have Huntington's disease, but Huntington's disease will remain a big part of my life as long as other family members are at risk or gene positive.

Belonging to an HD family is a lifelong experience. Long before I heard of Huntington's disease, I witnessed it firsthand. I never got to know or understand who my dad really was before Huntington's disease gradually took him away. I saw my brother struggle with symptoms that had no explanation. Now, I know what it's like to be at risk for a fatal genetic disorder and feel the intense worry that I may have passed it on to my kids. It is hard for me to talk about my experiences, and I find it difficult to describe Huntington's disease in a way that captures its complexity. I know how isolating this can be.

By not knowing we are an HD family, however, I didn't experience what it's like to grow up and enter adulthood wondering if I'm gene positive. I didn't have to think about a future in which I might develop Huntington's disease until long after I had already made career and family decisions. I had an easier time making these life decisions than my brother's at-risk kids do now that they're young adults. Huntington's disease factors into every major decision they make, and my family and I continue to worry about their futures. As my brother's symptoms continue to progress, I'm experiencing Huntington's disease in a new way. I'm learning what it's like to witness a loved one disappear slowly, and soon I'll witness my brother's final stage of Huntington's disease. This is uncharted territory for me and my family.

Sharing the HD story

Since my brother's diagnosis, I've had to explain Huntington's disease and my own HD experience many times. It's a rare disease, so few people have heard of it. There is always so much more to tell than what I can share in a quick conversation, so I often feel like my explanations fall short, even after 10 years of practice. I find myself wishing others were as familiar with Huntington's disease as they are with Alzheimer's or Parkinson's, so I didn't have to give a lesson in HD 101 before I could help somebody understand what it's like to belong to an HD family.

One of the best ways to understand the impacts of Huntington's disease is through personal accounts, but my own account is just one small piece of a complex story. I want people to know the bigger HD story, so I reached out to the HD community to find people willing to share how Huntington's disease impacts them. I talked with as many people as I could to capture a wide variety of experiences. As I spoke with people from around the world, I was struck by how quickly I was

Livable Lives Storytellers Around the World

My interviews took me (virtually) around the world to talk with people in 10 different countries!

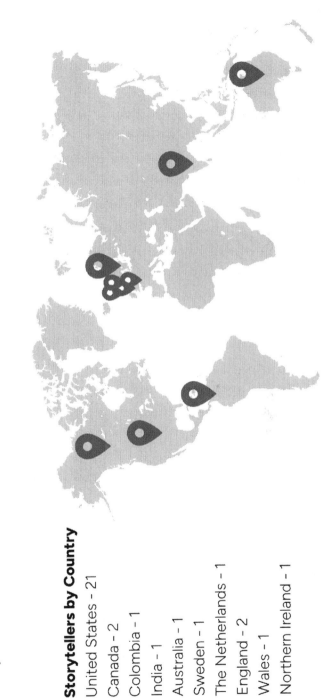

Storytellers by Country

United States – 21
Canada – 2
Colombia – 1
India – 1
Australia – 1
Sweden – 1
The Netherlands – 1
England – 2
Wales – 1
Northern Ireland – 1

drawn into each of their narratives. Every story was unique, each conversation provided another piece of the puzzle, and my understanding of Huntington's disease grew.

I began conversations with a list of questions that matched my ideas of what it means to belong to an HD family, but it didn't take long to realize that when I gave people space to tell their story how they wanted to tell it, they revealed experiences and thoughts I hadn't considered. Most conversations lasted about two hours, but several were much longer, and there were times when I barely spoke a word. I sensed an urgency from those sharing their stories – especially from those who know they are gene positive and want to share their experiences and document who they are before they become too symptomatic to do so.

Some people approached our conversation as an opportunity to continue their own efforts as public advocates for the HD community. Others saw the conversation as a chance to talk openly about Huntington's disease, sometimes for the first time. I talked with people who are at risk, gene positive, and gene negative. I talked with family members, researchers, and care providers. In all, I spoke with more than 30 people from 10 countries across five continents.

As you read their stories and mine, you'll notice similarities and differences. Most people mention how they first learned about Huntington's disease and its genetic component. They describe loved ones before and after HD symptoms set in. They talk about their own approach to the genetic testing decision and how the disease has affected their life choices. Some of their families talk openly about Huntington's disease while others do not.

Each story highlights a specific aspect of Huntington's disease, but each person's full story is included to provide a complete picture of their unique HD experience. You'll learn how each person copes and what they do to create their own version of a livable life while facing this devastating disease. You'll come to understand why it can be difficult to talk about Huntington's disease, but also why it is important to encourage ongoing conversations. Together, our stories reveal the complexities of Huntington's disease and its impact on families and individuals.

I think often about each of the people I spoke with. I wonder how their lives have changed since we last talked. Many of them laughed or cried as they told their stories, or the tone of their voices changed as they talked about their loved ones and their own wishes for the future. Like me, they want their stories to help increase awareness and understanding of Huntington's disease. So, I invite you to get to know this community that is often misunderstood and overlooked – a community full of diverse voices and experiences with valuable lessons to share.

HD 101

Huntington's disease made a grand entrance into my family's story when my brother was diagnosed 10 years ago. We went from knowing nothing about a disease that has an oversized impact on our lives to trying to learn as much as possible so we could understand what we were facing. I quickly learned that Huntington's disease is genetic, neurodegenerative, and incurable. A person with Huntington's disease experiences physical and cognitive decline along with significant changes in mood and behavior. Over time, a person with Huntington's disease loses the ability to walk, talk, and participate in daily life. But Huntington's disease is so much more than that.

I set out to write a comprehensive description of Huntington's disease, but it quickly turned into list after list of physical, cognitive, and behavioral symptoms. It often felt like I was adding to the inventory of potential symptoms with every description I encountered. The more I read, the more complicated explaining Huntington's disease seemed to become. I felt bogged down by the enormity of the task I had set for myself. Instead of explaining Huntington's disease as a list of symptoms, a better place to start might be sharing some of the impacts of Huntington's disease.

Certain things stand out to me. People with Huntington's disease experience extensive decline during the prime years of life. HD families face periodic crises, and the disease has a large impact on family relationships. Individuals and families experience loss after loss. When I first learned about Huntington's disease, I thought that if I was gene positive, I would become unrecognizable and unknowable and unlovable. I had a deep fear of losing myself and drifting inward and away from those I love. I struggled to imagine anything good about a life in which I had Huntington's disease. I didn't get tested right away because I wasn't ready to accept a positive result as my reality. I couldn't see anything *livable* about that version of my future.

Ten years later, I now know a life with Huntington's disease can include happiness and our family will make the most of our situation. We have a lot to be grateful for. But I also know Huntington's disease creates a kind of loss that runs deep. There's more to this loss than my brother's decline and our family's heartache. Huntington's disease takes away many of the things that *could-have-been* – the family we could have had growing up, the plans and memories we could have made with our loved ones, the future we could have looked forward to, and perhaps most importantly, the version of our loved ones we could have had and would love to continue to have in our lives. I am certain that a world in which my brother could have existed without Huntington's disease truly would have been a better one.

By far, other people's stories have helped me understand Huntington's disease in a way that clinical descriptions have not; and yet, a basic understanding of the disease's pattern of inheritance, symptoms, and history is essential to grasping the impact of Huntington's disease on families and individuals. So, let's dive in.

Genetics

Huntington's disease is caused by a single mutation in a single gene

– called the huntingtin gene – so it is often used as an example in biology classes when it's time to learn about genetics. Simply put, Huntington's disease occurs when a genetic mutation causes there to be too many repeats of the letters C-A-G in the DNA code of the huntingtin gene. When there are too many CAG repeats on the huntingtin gene, the brain produces a toxic form of the huntingtin protein that clumps together and prevents normal nerve cell function. Over time, many areas of the brain are affected, and brain cells die off.

We all have two copies of every gene – including the huntingtin gene – and we all inherit one copy of every gene from each of our parents. A parent who carries the mutation that causes Huntington's disease can pass on their normal copy of the huntingtin gene or their expanded copy – the one with too many CAG repeats. If a child inherits the expanded copy, they will develop Huntington's disease. If a child inherits the normal copy, they will not develop Huntington's disease. Therefore, every naturally conceived child of a parent with Huntington's disease has a 50-50 chance of inheriting it.

A person's HD gene status indicates whether they know if they have the expanded gene that causes Huntington's disease. If a person knows they might have inherited Huntington's disease, but they do not definitively know if they have the expanded gene, they are *at risk*. If they receive a positive genetic test or a clinical diagnosis, they are *gene positive*. If they, or their at-risk parent, receives a negative genetic test, they are *gene negative*.

A genetic test result for Huntington's disease includes two CAG repeat numbers. One shows the number of CAG repeats in the huntingtin gene inherited from the mother, and the other is the number of repeats in the huntingtin gene inherited from the father. CAG repeat numbers fall into four categories:

- People whose CAG repeat numbers are both *26 or less* are gene negative and will not develop Huntington's disease.
- People with a CAG repeat *between 27 and 35* are gene negative and will not develop Huntington's disease, but their children could potentially inherit a longer CAG repeat that puts them at higher risk

of developing Huntington's disease.
- Some people with a CAG repeat *between 36 and 39* will develop Huntington's disease while others will not, something that is called reduced penetrance.
- Everyone with a CAG repeat of *40 or more* is gene positive and will develop Huntington's disease.

My CAG repeat numbers are 13 and 18 – both normal – so I will never have Huntington's disease, and I cannot pass it on to my kids. My brother's CAG repeat numbers are 19 and 43, indicating he inherited a shorter normal copy from our mom and a longer mutated copy from our dad. His kids each have a 50-50 chance that they inherited the expanded gene from him.

The CAG repeat can increase in length when it is passed to the next generation, especially if it is inherited from a father. Longer CAG repeats are correlated with earlier disease onset and faster progression. People who develop Huntington's disease as an adult typically have a CAG repeat number between 40 and 50. When a CAG repeat becomes very long – typically 60 or higher – the disease can begin during childhood and is called Juvenile Huntington's disease.

While people with a CAG repeat in the 27 to 35 range will not develop Huntington's disease themselves, it is possible their children will inherit a CAG repeat that is longer and potentially long enough to cause Huntington's disease, perhaps becoming the first in their family to have the disease. This is called a new mutation to Huntington's disease.

Only some people with a CAG repeat between 36 and 39 will develop Huntington's disease. This range is often referred to as the *gray area*. In this case, a person might go through the stressful genetic testing process and still not know if they will develop Huntington's disease. Uncertainty is their only certainty. Individuals in this range who do develop Huntington's disease may have symptom onset later in life or develop less severe symptoms than those with a CAG repeat of 40 or more. Very few people receive a genetic test result in this range, so there are few resources tailored to their unique experience and needs.

It is important to note that the 50-50 chance of inheriting Huntington's disease does not mean that half of the children in an HD family will develop the disease. These 50-50 odds can be compared to tossing a coin. Each time a coin is tossed, there is a 50-50 chance it will land on heads. The HD status of one child has no bearing on the status of their brothers or sisters. Each child has their own 50-50 chance of inheriting Huntington's disease – their own coin to toss. It is possible for all offspring of a gene-positive parent to inherit Huntington's disease, and it is also possible for none of them to inherit it, but the outcome is usually somewhere in between.

Inheritance is not tied in any way to sex, race, or ethnicity, though there is a higher prevalence of the disease in North America, Australia, and Western Europe. In the United States, it is estimated that more than 40,000 people have symptomatic Huntington's disease, and another 200,000 are at risk.

Gene status

If you belong to an HD family, your gene status may be a central part of your identity. People who are at risk for Huntington's disease may have a constant, low-grade anxiety about whether they carry the expanded gene, what that means for the future, and whether they should seek out predictive genetic testing. Sometimes, people are convinced they have Huntington's disease before getting tested, even in the absence of symptoms. Once an at-risk person is much older than their HD parent was at symptom onset, they may start to relax a little, but there is always the possibility they are gene positive and will have a later age of onset. Only a small percentage of people seek out genetic testing if symptoms are not present, so some people remain technically at risk their entire lives.

A person may learn they are gene positive before symptoms appear if they seek out predictive genetic testing and receive a positive result.

At this point, they enter a period of limbo in which symptoms are not yet present, but symptom development is inevitable and may feel imminent. Symptom searching is common among people who are at risk or gene positive. It is easy to interpret stumbles or normal reactions to everyday stress as early signs of disease. Getting angry during a disagreement or feeling anxious about the future could be interpreted as symptomatic changes in mood. These could be normal reactions, or they could, in fact, be early signs.

Alternatively, a person may not learn they are gene positive until symptoms appear and a clinical examination or genetic test confirms their diagnosis. Common stresses among those who are gene positive include worries about burdening others as the disease progresses, guilt over the possibility of passing the expanded gene to the next generation, experiencing unkindness and ignorance from others who don't understand HD symptoms, and losing income when working is no longer possible. Symptom onset and progression are devastating for both the gene-positive person and their loved ones.

There are two ways for a person to definitively know they are gene negative and do not carry the expanded HD gene. If an at-risk parent tests negative, then their children are also gene negative. Or an at-risk person can go through the predictive genetic testing process themselves and receive a negative test result. People who test negative but had prepared to receive a positive result may have trouble re-orienting their life to include a healthy future. Some experience a sense of loss that's hard to explain, and many feel a sense of survivor's guilt.

HD symptoms

While inheritance of Huntington's disease is straightforward, its symptoms are not. The disease can look different from person to person, which becomes clear when you meet or hear stories from multiple people with the disease. Symptoms typically appear when a person is between 30 and 50 years old, though they can develop at any age. Doctors may misdiagnose cases in children or the elderly, thinking the person is too young or too old to develop Huntington's disease. In general, a longer CAG repeat is associated with an earlier age of symptom onset and more severe disease. However, there is not a one-to-one correlation, so members of the same family can have the same CAG repeat length and still develop symptoms at different ages or with different degrees of severity. They may even have different collections of symptoms.

Subtle cognitive and behavioral symptoms often appear before physical symptoms, but there is no pre-determined order, and a person's collection of symptoms can change over the course of the disease. Early symptoms appear slowly and may not be recognized initially as Huntington's disease. A person may seem more confrontational than normal or have trouble completing tasks that are normally easy for them. Such changes can be confusing or aggravating for family members. In my conversations, I heard over and over that loved ones with Huntington's disease started acting out of character early in the course of their disease – their behavior didn't make sense. This matches my own experience of my dad's behavior when I was in elementary school. He wasn't himself.

A person with Huntington's disease can have any mix of the disease's physical, cognitive, and behavioral symptoms in varying degrees of severity – from mild to quite severe. Ultimately, symptom variability is captured in a common saying in the HD world: "If you've met one person with Huntington's disease, you've met one person with Huntington's disease." The following is a review of many, but not all, of the symptoms a person with Huntington's disease may experience.

Physical Symptoms

Huntington's disease is a movement disorder, and chorea is its most recognizable symptom. About 90 percent of people with Huntington's disease have these involuntary movements that often start in the eyes, fingers, toes, and tongue, and later include the arms, legs, and torso. Chorea looks like a continual cycle of large jerky movements and unusual facial grimaces. It would be easy to think a person with Huntington's disease is impaired by alcohol or drugs rather than a neurological condition, and it is common for people with the disease to be stopped by the police for this reason.

Now that I know what chorea looks like, it's hard to miss. A few years before my brother was diagnosed, my brother's son brought a college friend home for dinner with the family. My brother's chorea was immediately recognizable to the friend who knew someone with Huntington's disease. When the friend later asked if my brother had Huntington's disease, it seemed like a strange question. Huntington's disease was not on my family's radar, nor did we know anything about it or what it looked like. After my brother's diagnosis, however, I went to an HD support group and was struck by how much one of the attendees reminded me of my brother, especially the way he moved. It was distinctive and unmistakable.

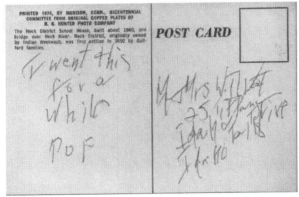

My grandpa's handwriting on this postcard reminds me of changes I saw in my brother's handwriting as his symptoms progressed.

As chorea becomes more pronounced and less controlled, a person with Huntington's disease begins to experience an unsteady gait and a lack of coordination and balance. They eventually lose the ability to walk. As chorea progresses, movements can result in unintentional harm to self or others or physical damage to a home or facility. My brother has broken several wheelchairs, he wore through the linoleum floor in his kitchen by moving his chair back and forth repeatedly, and his shoes wear out quickly even though he uses a wheelchair.

A weakening of muscles in the face and tongue results in two other common HD symptoms: slurred speech and difficulty swallowing. Slurred speech makes it hard for people with Huntington's disease to communicate with others, which can be frustrating and isolating. Difficulty swallowing increases the risks of choking and aspirating food or liquids. Choking incidents can be traumatizing for a person with Huntington's disease and for family members who witness severe incidents.

Many people with Huntington's disease lose a lot of weight due to increased metabolism, constant movements, and difficulty eating – getting food from the plate to the mouth successfully can be a challenge. Insomnia and sleep disturbances can cause a person with Huntington's disease to flip their sleep schedule and begin sleeping during the day, resulting in poor sleep that can aggravate other symptoms. Finally, pain is a symptom that is reported by many people with Huntington's disease, but it is not well researched and may be insufficiently treated.

Cognitive symptoms

Huntington's disease causes cognitive impairment that affects how a person interprets and responds to the world around them. Cognitive losses accumulate as Huntington's disease progresses, and family members report that the loved one they once knew slowly disappears. Despite this decline, a person with Huntington's disease remains aware of their surroundings and can understand what people say to them even in the last stage of the disease when they are no longer able to communicate.

A declining ability to process information results in slower thinking, confusion, and a loss of mental flexibility, all of which make it more challenging to complete tasks and manage self-care. It becomes more difficult to participate in conversation as it takes longer to process and answer questions. Eventually, a person with Huntington's disease loses the ability to talk, due to a mix of cognitive and physical changes.

Cognitive changes can also include impaired judgment, compromised decision-making skills, and an inability to reason or be reasoned with. Add in impulsivity, and a person with Huntington's disease can easily find themselves in problematic situations.

An impaired ability to understand their own and others' emotions combined with difficulty expressing feelings can make it hard for people with Huntington's disease to form and maintain interpersonal relationships. A formerly engaged and loving family member may lack empathy or disregard the emotional needs of loved ones, for example. This does not mean, however, that people with Huntington's disease don't feel emotions. Decreased self-awareness results in an interesting phenomenon. Many people with Huntington's disease have something called anosognosia, which is an inability to recognize one's own physical, cognitive, or behavioral symptoms. Some people are not aware that they have chorea or impaired judgment, for example, even if these symptoms are very apparent to others.

Behavioral Symptoms

Behavioral symptoms are often mentioned as the most challenging to cope with. While some people have mild behavioral symptoms, others have severe symptoms that can look like schizophrenia or bipolar disorder. Changes in mood can include depression, anxiety, irritability, extreme mood swings, and apathy. These behavioral changes can result in social withdrawal, not wanting to leave the house, and difficulty getting out of bed and ready for the day even when there is a desire to do so. It is important to note that some behavioral symptoms, like depression, are due to disease-related changes in the brain, not just a response to having a fatal disease.

Perseverative thinking and obsessive-compulsive disorder are common symptoms that can result in repetitive thoughts or behaviors, or unrelenting worry or fear. Controlling emotions and impulses becomes difficult for those with Huntington's disease, especially as it becomes harder to interpret the world around them. Unpredictable behavior, outbursts, and even sexual promiscuity are potential symptoms, as are inappropriate or irrational behaviors. Some people are easily irritated and prone to anger or aggression. Psychosis is less common, but some people do experience paranoia, hallucinations, or delusions.

An unfortunate reality for HD families is that people with Huntington's disease have a higher risk of suicide. Behavioral red flags that should not be ignored include thoughts about suicide or self-harm, aggressive behavior, alcohol or substance abuse, paranoid thoughts, and command hallucinations, which are auditory hallucinations that direct a person to do something or act in a certain way. HD families can get help by consulting with a medical provider, seeking emergency care, reaching out to an HD organization, or accessing a crisis hotline if their country has one.

Overall, people with Huntington's disease have symptoms that may seem strange to someone who doesn't know them. Their movements and behaviors draw attention; they might act in unpredictable and aggressive ways; and they may not have the cognitive ability to answer questions or show good judgment. Altogether, these symptoms set the stage for misunderstandings when out in public where symptoms are not recognized as signs of a neurological disorder. If a person with symptomatic Huntington's disease does not have support, or their behavioral symptoms are severe, they may fall through the cracks and not receive the care they need. They may disappear for days or longer, become homeless, or have interactions with the police.

Disease progression

Once symptoms appear, the duration of Huntington's disease can be anywhere from 10 to 25 years, or even longer. While diet and exercise cannot prevent a person from developing Huntington's disease, following a healthy lifestyle may have a positive influence on age of onset and disease progression. The progression of Huntington's disease is characterized by several stages, each lasting many years. Transitions from one stage to the next are slow and somewhat ambiguous, as each person's progression may look different based on their own collection and severity of symptoms. Some HD symptoms can be managed by medication or a variety of therapies – like physical, occupational, and speech therapy – but there is currently nothing available to prevent, slow, or reverse the disease's progressive physical, cognitive, and behavioral decline.

Huntington's disease progresses through several stages. When a person is gene positive but does not yet have measurable symptoms, they are *presymptomatic*. A person enters the *prodromal period* when they begin having subtle cognitive and behavioral symptoms. Once a person starts to exhibit chorea, they enter the *early stage* of Huntington's disease. Chorea typically needs to be present to receive a clinical diagnosis of disease onset. Again, chorea is the involuntary movements of the face, limbs, and torso that are characteristic of the disease. Changes in coordination and an impaired ability to problem solve may appear in this earliest stage. People may also begin having depression, irritability, and sleep disturbances. In most cases, a person in this stage can still function fully at work and home.

In the *middle stage*, impairments are more pronounced, and a person loses the ability to hold down a job, manage finances, and contribute to household responsibilities. Some people leave their jobs of their own accord, but many are let go by their employers. In this stage, people can continue to care for themselves and perform normal daily tasks – like eating and personal hygiene – but they may require some assistance. If they have chorea, it will be much more noticeable, and voluntary motor movements will become more difficult. This is the period when most people lose the ability to drive. Problems with balance, speaking, swallowing, and maintaining weight may appear, and problem solving becomes more challenging. This is a period of decreasing independence and increasing reliance on assistance from others.

In the *late stage*, chorea may be severe, or it may be replaced by muscle rigidity, involuntary muscle contractions, and slowing or freezing of movements. At this point, a person with Huntington's disease will need assistance with all activities of daily living. They are likely to become nonverbal and bedridden and may require tube feeding. If psychiatric symptoms are present, they become harder to detect and treat because of impaired communication. As the disease continues to progress, a person is likely to need professional, around-the-clock nursing care. Most people die from complications of the disease, such as choking, aspiration pneumonia, or malnutrition. It is important to plan for this last stage to best meet the needs and wishes of the patient. Creating a living will and having early conversations can help family members understand what is important and tolerable to our loved ones at the end of their lives.

A brief history

Over the last 150 years, there have been many steps toward a better understanding of Huntington's disease. Before there was a scientific description of the disease, people with unusual movements might have been diagnosed with the *magrums* or *St. Vitus's dance*. These were catch-all terms for a variety of movement disorders that were not yet understood. In 1872, Dr. George Huntington published a complete description of Huntington's disease, including its pattern of inheritance, in his article, *On Chorea*. He was only 22 years old and had just received his medical degree. He had encountered people with Huntington's disease while growing up in East Hampton, New York, where his father and grandfather had both served as physicians to a concentrated number of HD families. Dr. Huntington's description soon became the standard definition, and the disease was later named after him.

A significant breakthrough in understanding the cause of Huntington's disease came in 1983, when a team of researchers at Massachusetts General Hospital narrowed the location of the huntingtin gene to chromosome 4. This discovery allowed development of the first predictive genetic test for Huntington's disease. It used a technique called linkage analysis that required DNA samples from multiple family members, both affected and unaffected. Dr. Nancy Wexler, who belongs to an HD family herself, was a member of this team.

Dr. Wexler devoted her career to HD research and led another team of researchers that pinpointed the exact genetic mutation that causes Huntington's disease in 1993. To do this, Dr. Wexler's team spent weeks at a time visiting remote Venezuelan communities near Lake Maracaibo where there is a very high concentration of HD families. Over two decades, the team collected thousands of blood samples and mapped HD lineages for thousands of people across 10 generations. Their discovery allows individuals to do direct genetic testing without needing DNA samples from other family members. HD researchers continue to advance our knowledge of the pathology of Huntington's disease but have yet to develop a disease-modifying treatment or cure. Currently, the only available treatments are drugs that lessen chorea and manage psychiatric symptoms.

Huntington's disease has a long history of stigmatization, but in the United States, the eugenics movement of the early 20th century was particularly harmful and silenced many families. The eugenics movement advocated selective breeding and sterilization to increase characteristics regarded as desirable and decrease those considered undesirable. The Eugenics Record Office (ERO) served as a national clearinghouse for data collected on American families. Targeted populations included immigrants, non-whites, the poor, and those who had mental illness, disabilities, or diseases like Huntington's disease. By 1938, tens of thousands of Americans had been involuntarily sterilized.

In the United States, eugenics became discredited and the ERO closed in 1939 after the ideas promoted by American eugenics were adopted by Nazi Germany, but the damage was already done. This detrimental period increased stigma and negative perceptions of Huntington's disease and contributed to many families keeping the disease a family secret. Some HD families hid family members with noticeable symptoms or confined them to remote parts of the home to protect them.

Stigmatization of Huntington's disease is lessening but hasn't gone away, and it remains pervasive in some countries.

Several organizations work to improve the lives of HD families. Famed folk singer and songwriter, Woodie Guthrie, died of Huntington's disease in 1967. That same year, his widow, Marjorie Guthrie, helped establish the Huntington's Disease Society of America (HDSA). Several years later, she helped establish the International Huntington Association. These organizations, and many others around the world, are dedicated to raising awareness, providing support, improving care, and promoting research.

More recently, the advent of social media and youth-centered organizations – like the Huntington's Disease Youth Organization (HDYO), HDSA's National Youth Alliance, and others – are fostering a new generation determined to reduce stigma and connect with others in the HD community. These changes mark a paradigm shift in which advocacy is moving to center stage to replace secrecy and fear. While stigma still exists and not all families and individuals are comfortable talking about Huntington's disease, these changes are creating a sense of community in the HD world – a significant change from the days when many individuals and families felt they were facing this disease alone.

RESOURCES

Worldwide, there are many HD organizations that provide information, resources, and support for the HD community. Many of these organizations also provide research updates and opportunities to connect with others. Websites for local, regional, national, and international HD organizations can be found online with a simple search, and websites for HDYO (hdyo.org) and the International Huntington Association (huntington-disease.org) provide links to country-specific websites. A selection of HD organizations is listed below.

Selected International Organizations
- Huntington's Disease Youth Organization
- International Huntington Association
- European Huntington's Disease Network
- Help4HD International

National Organizations for *Livable Lives* Storytellers' Countries
- Huntington's Disease Society of America
- Huntington Society of Canada
- Huntington's Australia
- Huntington Disease Society of India
- Fundacion Huntington do Colombia
- Riksförbundet Huntingtons Sjukdom (Sweden)
- Vereniging van Huntington (The Netherlands)
- Huntington's Disease Association (England and Wales)
- Huntington's Disease Association Northern Ireland

Selected Youth & Young Adult Organizations
- Huntington's Disease Youth Organization (International)
- HDSA's National Youth Alliance (United States)
- Young People Affected by Huntington's Disease (Canada)

Selected HD Foundations and Nonprofits
- The Hidden No More Foundation (raises awareness to reduce stigma)
- Hereditary Disease Foundation (supports research)
- HD Reach (serves families in North Carolina and beyond)
- HelpCureHD (helps couples in the United States and Canada have HD-free babies)

A FAMILY DISEASE

Even though we didn't know we were an HD family until 10 years ago, Huntington's disease has been part of my life since I was seven years old, and I've seen its impact on my family from one generation to the next. I saw my grandpa in the final stage of the disease when he was bedridden and no longer able to communicate. I experienced my family's struggles when my dad and brother each exhibited a confusing mix of symptoms. My brother may be slowly transitioning to the last stage of Huntington's disease, and I see the emotional toll on his wife and kids. I also see my brother's kids grapple with their at-risk status as they travel alongside their dad in his decline. It's the same path followed by many HD families.

The HD story repeats itself generation after generation, so HD families face a perpetual cycle of disease and loss until there comes a day – for some families – that they are lucky enough that no one else carries the expanded gene. This can happen, but it is all too rare. Instead of wondering *if* another family member will be affected, families are faced with wondering *who* will be next. At-risk family members witness the effects of Huntington's disease on relatives before potentially developing the disease themselves. People in multiple generations, and multiple people in each generation, may be symptomatic at the same time. The

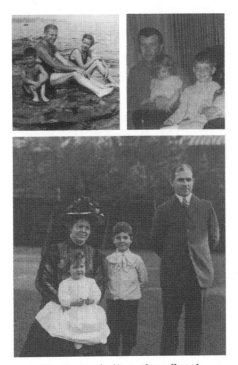

Huntington's disease has affected my family for multiple generations.

slow progression of the disease means families are in the thick of caring for loved ones with Huntington's disease for years, or more likely, decades. Families live through the trauma of loss after loss, only to do it all over again.

When telling our HD stories, most of us start in one of two places: we either describe our family tree of relatives with Huntington's disease, or we tell how we learned about Huntington's disease for the first time. We give an accounting of where Huntington's disease came from and how it arrived at our doorstep. The family nature of Huntington's disease is always apparent. Having a family disease sets your family apart from others. There are constant reminders of what could have been, and there is no chance of a normal path through life. It's a lifelong journey that affects the entire family. These may seem like broad overarching statements, but they ring true for those of us who live this life. This is our reality.

Multiple family members are affected

In my lifetime, only one family member in each generation has had Huntington's disease. If we had multiple family members in each generation, the losses and challenges we experience now would be compounded. At the time my brother was diagnosed, it was possible that 10 of my family members could have inherited Huntington's disease – three in my generation, and seven in the next. What if all of us had been gene positive? With each additional gene-positive family member, we would experience more disease, more decline, and more loss, and there would be greater impact on family members' wellbeing, social isolation, and finances.

Many HD families have more gene-positive family members than my family does. Jim, from Illinois, can count more than 30 family members with the disease in recent generations, including his mom. Since genetic testing became available, Jim is the only person in his family to test negative, and his children are the first family members since 1900 to be born knowing they will not develop Huntington's disease. Several people in Jim's family, including his siblings, have not been tested but have classic HD symptoms. "People just keep falling off like leaves," he said. Jim sometimes envies families where the disease progresses quickly. "In my family, it seems like a 40-year problem. It's nonstop; there's no closure."

Jim has been surrounded by Huntington's disease his whole life. When he attended an HD conference, he commented to a friend that he felt very relaxed in a room full of people with Huntington's disease. "People were pulling the tablecloths off, and food was going everywhere. I felt right at home," he said. "How weird is that? But for me, it was a comforting feeling." Despite Jim's comfort with being around people with Huntington's disease, belonging to an HD family has had a significant impact on his wellbeing. He's only recently been able to talk about his experiences. "I was muted for so long because I couldn't talk about it. I don't think I could have done this 10 years ago, five years ago, even," he said. "I think people are sick of letting the disease win. My words right now are a battle against the disease."

As a child, Jim frequently accompanied his mom and grandma to the VA hospital to visit his grandpa who had Huntington's disease. Jim has good memories of these peaceful visits. They would have a picnic, and Jim would putt a golf ball around a small putting green. His grandpa would tell him extraordinary stories about his adventures, like his secret mission to China. This made sense to Jim because there were signs of the military all around the VA hospital, but in reality, his grandpa was never part of a secret mission.

Jim would tell his mom and grandma, "You guys don't even know grandpa. He's a secret agent, and he's awesome! He's just trying to keep you guys safe." When these visits came to an end, however, Jim's grandpa returned to the hospital's psychiatric ward. His grandpa's early HD symptoms were attributed to PTSD due to his time serving in the military during WWII, and he received several other misdiagnoses, including schizophrenia, before doctors properly diagnosed him with Huntington's disease. Despite his grandpa's delusional thinking, Jim was never scared of his grandpa or his grandpa's disease.

One of Jim's aunts had similar delusions, which Jim noticed when he traveled with her. She would hide from airport workers she thought were undercover agents. "I can't imagine that paranoia side of it," he said. This aunt has passed away, and his other aunt is now bedridden and no longer able to speak. When Jim visits her, he likes to reminisce to make her laugh. "If you saw her, you would think she's not there anymore, but she will die laughing remembering a story from 25 or 30 years ago," he said. "I think that's what people don't understand about this disease. The brain still works; the memory's still there." Jim thought his aunt would have passed away long ago, but his uncle thinks she holds on because she enjoys seeing her grandkids. "It's beautiful, in a way, to see how sick she is, and she's willing to still fight like that to be alive. She's still a grandma, you know."

Jim understood Huntington's disease at a young age. His family talked openly about the disease, but he was also intensely curious and a quick learner. He wanted to know everything. "I was that kid who was in the medical research section of the library at 10 years old rather than the picture book section," he said. Even with this knowledge, Jim was often confused by his mom's HD symptoms. Over the years, Jim's mom disappeared on numerous occasions. She would head for Canada without telling anyone. Hours later, she would get scared and call home before driving back in tears.

At times, Jim's mom seemed gregarious, but then her demeanor would change suddenly. "She would snap into that authoritative weird person," he said. "You didn't know what was happening hour-by-hour, day-by-day." Jim knew his mom's behavior was due to Huntington's disease, but it was still hard to be on the receiving end of her outbursts. There was no one to blame and nowhere to go. The unpredictability Jim experienced growing up in an HD family continues to make him uncomfortable in situations where there are a lot of unknowns.

Many of Jim's symptomatic family members are in denial about having Huntington's disease, which prevents them from getting the care and services they desperately need. "I have 30 people with this, right? Nobody can help anybody," he said. Surprisingly, Jim's dad is also in denial that Jim's mom has Huntington's disease. For years, Jim's dad has attributed her symptoms to menopause. When Jim was just 20 years old, he researched menopause and figured out his mom's symptoms didn't look anything like what other women experience. "Why does he think it's menopause? We saw 100 women that could have been in menopause, and there was one lady running around playing hide-and-seek with people, and that was Mom."

In recent years, Jim has removed himself from family interactions due to the negative impact of his mom's behavioral symptoms on their relationship. He still texts with family, but he doesn't see them in person. "I've learned that everybody has a point where they have to remove themselves, and that was one of the hardest things for me to do," he said. "It took me years, but that was very important to my psyche and wellbeing. I've removed myself from the negative aspects. I guess it's my choice now to be involved in the parts that I want to be involved in and to be an advocate for myself."

While Jim understands that others might question him for limiting interactions with his family, he knows he would have had his grandma's support. He was close to his grandma and even chose to spend time with her before hanging out with friends when he was in high school. When Jim asked his grandma how she navigated having family members with Huntington's disease, she said, "You just take care of you, Jim. I know that's hard to do, but take care of you; and then, when you can, use love to take care of others."

Jim admired his grandma's steadfast commitment to family members with Huntington's disease. After Jim's grandpa moved to the VA hospital, she called every day to see how he was doing, and for nearly 40 years, she drove long distances to visit him every weekend. Jim credits his grandma with holding the whole family together. Family ties have unraveled since she died and as family members' HD symptoms have progressed. Jim distinctly remembers a conversation he had with his grandma before she died. "The only thing I regret saying was, 'What if I'm the only one in this family that doesn't have this disease? What do you want me to do?'" he asked her. "And again, the answer from her was treat people with love, right?"

When asked what he wishes people outside the HD community knew, Jim immediately answered, "How hard it really is." This was followed by a long pause. He choked up as he continued. "That's an interesting question. I don't think people can understand it at all... ever. Think about your family members being prisoners of war, and you're right there watching, and you know they're dying from all the things they have wrong with them; and then, multiply that by exponential amounts, when you have people like me with multiple family members with it. Huntington's is like the silent problem. It's killing your family, and you can't even tell anybody about it, and nobody knows to ask." For Jim, one of the saddest parts of Huntington's disease is how much it has changed his mom's family as more and more relatives become symptomatic or pass away. When he spends time with extended family on his dad's side, things seem more normal, which makes Jim think even more about what his mom's family could have been like without the influence of Huntington's disease.

Before getting tested for Huntington's disease, Jim didn't care about much in life because he didn't think there was any chance that he was gene negative. As a kid, he engaged in reckless behaviors. "What did it matter?" he asked. "I wasn't rebellious. I just didn't care." One reason he thought he was gene positive was that he was angry all the time. "I don't want to say I was mad at people who were happy, but I was mad that people didn't have to deal with it." He later realized, "It was legit anger at this dumb disease. What I realized, too, is it's not anger; it's sadness. I would love to have my family, and I can't." When asked why he got tested if he didn't care, Jim said, "Because I wanted to care. Does that make sense? I thought I didn't care because I thought I had it."

When Jim's genetic counselor told him he was gene negative, his immediate response was, "Say that again?" He didn't believe it; he thinks he asked the genetic counselor to repeat his result five times. Jim struggled after testing negative. He remembers the exact moment – six months later – when his constant thoughts about Huntington's disease ceased. "I remember driving on the highway, and it just stopped... Almost like a click... My brain went quiet. I realized what it was, and it was a wonderful feeling, and then a weird feeling, like a sad feeling. I can't believe I'd been thinking about it that much."

Jim's life continues to be touched by Huntington's disease even though he and his children are gene negative. The worst part for Jim is seeing the disease impact so many of his family members. "I am going to watch everybody else leave," he said. "I'll have to redefine what it means to me to be a family, and what a birthday party means to my child. Grandma and Grandpa aren't going to be there. Aunts and uncles won't be there."

Jim finds it interesting that there are so many unique experiences of Huntington's disease. "It's a disease caused by genetic repeats, but the story is not repetitive," he said. "I see that as an amazing part of the disease." One reason the story is not repetitive is that all family members, including those who do not have Huntington's disease, are impacted by belonging to an HD family. Spouses, parents, and children of people with Huntington's disease add their own perspective to the collective HD story.

A spouse's perspective

Researchers have found that a spouse or partner experiences as much distress over a gene-positive test result as the gene carrier themselves. Even though my brother had been having symptoms for years, having a definitive HD diagnosis changed everything for him and his wife and tore their world apart. I have immense admiration for my sister-in-law – beyond what I can ever express in words. I appreciate the love and care and respect she shows for my brother. After his diagnosis, she continued to include him in family decisions and considered him as a co-parent and life partner as long as he was able. She continually advocates on his behalf with nonfamily caregivers and doctors. I love that she bought a two-person recliner for his room so they can sit together to watch a movie when she visits him at his group home. When she says she feels guilty for not doing enough – which is not true – or for wishing my brother didn't have to go through this, I do my best to console and support her, but it never feels like enough. There's nothing I can fix.

My sister-in-law did not have to contemplate having Huntington's disease herself, but that doesn't make her life any easier. She had to navigate accessing federal and state disability and health benefits for my brother while protecting their financial assets, and she gradually became a single parent of sorts. She feels the pressure of holding everything together while experiencing the gradual loss of her spouse. At the same time, she knows she may also lose one or more of their kids to the disease. She never imagined this would be her life when she and my brother got married.

My sister-in-law has had to make major decisions related to my brother's health and wellbeing, often with little guidance about how to choose the best way forward. She provides the type of safety net that is essential for someone with Huntington's disease when they are no longer able to care for themselves. My mom did the same for my dad. If my brother or dad had been on their own, they would not have been able to take care of themselves, and they could have ended up homeless or at the mercy of anyone who crossed their paths. They were lucky to have had spouses by their side along with a support network of family members.

The arrival of Huntington's disease in any relationship marks the loss of a normal future together. Many spouses and partners feel socially isolated as they face a disease that few people understand, and they are less likely than their gene-positive spouse or partner to seek out support groups and other types of support. There is a loss of intimacy and companionship as a spousal relationship changes from one of caring partners to a relationship between a caregiver and patient.

A spouse's caregiving responsibilities may extend to multiple generations of an HD family, including their gene-positive spouse or partner, the HD parent of their spouse or partner, and any of their children who develop Huntington's disease. They may even care for multiple family members at the same time. Many marriages do not survive Huntington's disease, and some end before an HD diagnosis explains behaviors that contributed to its breakdown. Many ex-spouses, however, continue to provide some level of care for their gene-positive partner after a marriage or relationship dissolves.

Spouses and partners face an endless stream of medical, financial, parenting, and other crises. When I talked with Zoey, she had recently gone through a period of crisis when her husband, Clive, moved to a nursing home for residents with significant needs. Zoey lives in England with their two children, ages 10 and 14. Zoey and the kids are adjusting to a new rhythm, one in which home life is no longer dominated by Huntington's disease. About her husband, Zoey said, "I'm not really his wife anymore. It's just me and the children now. It's bizarre."

Zoey didn't know anything about Huntington's disease when she met Clive, and neither did he – not until Clive's mother was diagnosed. For several years, Clive's mother had symptoms her doctors attributed to dementia. As other symptoms appeared, however, her doctors considered other causes and eventually diagnosed her with Huntington's disease. Clive decided to get tested soon after his mother's diagnosis and learned he also carries the expanded gene. "The world sort of crashed down," Zoey said. "It was very stressful and very heartbreaking. We were like, 'It's gonna happen in the future, so let's just move on.' We went traveling all over the place and just enjoyed life." Clive told Zoey she didn't have to stay with him, but she didn't want to leave. "I loved him," she said. "It would have been hard to walk away from this close loving relationship, you know?" That was 20 years ago.

When Zoey and Clive decided to have children, they conceived naturally and went through prenatal genetic testing at about 10 weeks into each pregnancy. Zoey's first pregnancy was terminated via abortion after the fetus tested positive for Huntington's disease, but the next two pregnancies gave them two gene-negative children. "We wanted to stop Huntington's in its tracks," she said. "It's really controversial for some people, but I don't regret it. It was tough, but now we have two healthy children who don't have the expanded gene, so that's the best thing ever."

Zoey thinks her children are doing well despite the progression of their dad's disease. The kids have known about Huntington's disease for a long time, and Zoey continues to have open and honest conversations with them. The kids will never truly know their dad, but Zoey has worked hard to be sure they have good memories of him. "Clive wanted a family. He was great with kids when he could be, and it was lovely," she said. "He loved them. We packed in a lot of family holidays for making memories. That was the goal: get the kids to remember what they can of their dad."

Clive started having early HD symptoms a decade ago. He became depressed and lost his job. He no longer had a laidback personality, and he had trouble completing tasks. When Zoey consulted with the

Huntington's Disease Association, she was told these were classic symptoms. Clive, however, thought nothing was wrong; he didn't even see his own movements. When a doctor asked him to sit in a chair and watch his body for 20 seconds, it was obvious to the doctor and Zoey that Clive had chorea. When the time was up, Clive said, "I told you I don't move."

When Clive eventually accepted that he was symptomatic, he started meeting regularly with a team of specialists at the local HD clinic. Zoey was impressed with the level of care he received. Clive would listen to this team when he wouldn't listen to her, so Zoey relied on them to help with difficult conversations. When she became worried about the safety of his driving, she worked with the team to tell Clive he needed to take a driving test. He lost his driver's license but continued to be tempted to drive. "That was awful," Zoey said. "And then, luckily, the car broke down, so I purposefully didn't get that fixed. It sat on the drive broken. We left it there for quite a while."

Clive maintained his physical strength by biking. "Honestly, he cycled better than he walked," Zoey said. She got him a lifeline pendant so she could track him when he was out on his bike. If he left home without her knowledge, the button was a lifesaver. She could speak to him directly through a speaker in the device to tell him to head for home. When it was no longer safe for Clive to go out on his own, Zoey told him the bike-lock key was lost and she was waiting for a new one to be delivered. He accepted that but continued to go out each day to look for the missing key.

While Clive has had mostly cognitive and psychiatric symptoms, he's had physical symptoms as well. His disease progressed gradually at first, but near the end of his time at home, he started to exhibit aggressive behaviors and required round-the-clock monitoring. Zoey relied heavily on support from family and friends who helped her take small breaks now and then. Eventually, Clive's symptoms worsened to the point that Zoey hired in-home caregivers to care for him while she worked. She continued to provide 100 percent of his care outside of her work hours.

Clive's behavioral symptoms included several obsessions, one of which was showering. Soon after finishing a shower, he would disappear to take another. "And then he got to the point where he couldn't turn the shower on," Zoey said. "He would come downstairs with shampoo on his head, and he was just oblivious." When Zoey would ask Clive about it, he would reply, "What shampoo are you talking about?" Another obsession was time. Clive fixated on whatever he thought he needed to do next and what time it needed to be done. If this happened near bedtime, it often meant he would be up all night.

Over time, Clive's speech became difficult to understand and his ability to swallow deteriorated. "His eating and swallowing went about four years ago," Zoey said. "That slowly led to coughing, sputtering, and then choking episodes. So frightening. He's choked and passed out in front of the kids." Zoey had to do the Heimlich maneuver on Clive at the dinner table one Christmas Day. Another time, she made a quick trip to the store and returned to find Clive choking on the floor. He now eats pureed foods but insists he doesn't want a feeding tube.

Clive has been admitted to the hospital several times for chest infections caused by aspiration, but emergency room visits triggered behavioral symptoms that became unmanageable. His last emergency room visit was very stressful. Being away from home and out of his routine made Clive confused and agitated. Hospital staff asked Zoey to leave, which made her uncomfortable. She was worried about Clive being on his own in a setting where people didn't understand Huntington's disease. As she left the hospital, she heard him urgently and anxiously repeat over and over, "My name is Clive, and I've got Huntington's disease... My name is Clive, and I've got Huntington's disease..." After that, Zoey worked with Clive's medical team to manage his medical needs without going to the hospital.

Clive now lives in a skilled nursing facility where one-on-one caregivers rotate every two hours due to the intensity of clients' needs. The day he was admitted to the nursing home was especially tough. Clive had no understanding of what was happening. "He was fine going in; he was fine seeing the people. That didn't bother him," Zoey said. "But things are locked because of people's needs. When we got in there, he said, 'The door's locking... The door's locking...' I was there 40 minutes, and he went absolutely ballistic. He went on a rampage; he was literally attacking them. I'd not seen that before. They were all geared up and trained in managing people at that level of behavior and doing the emergency restraints. I had to leave the building once it started because I was just in bits. I didn't want to see that." Zoey learned the next day that this went on for six hours. "I felt so bad," she said. "The guilt... What have I done to him?"

Zoey feels like Huntington's disease has been ever-present in her life since Clive tested positive. "You wake up with it every day," she said. "Even before he started having symptoms, it would be rare that I wasn't thinking about Huntington's disease. And then boom... There it is. You see your loved one – the love of your life – and now he's lost... There are constant losses." By the time Clive moved to the nursing home, Zoey no longer recognized him as the man she loved. For several years, she had only seen Clive as the person right in front of her, the one with symptomatic Huntington's disease.

Zoey became emotional as she explained how her perception of Clive changed after he moved to the nursing home. "Something in my brain filled with memories of him from before, like when we started out. It all came flooding in," she said. Zoey paused as she started to cry. "Suddenly, it's hitting home that he's extremely unwell. I can see that now, but I couldn't see it when I lived with him. He lost the ability to smile and laugh and have happiness quite a long time ago. It's so sad because he was the gentlest man."

Clive is still adjusting to the nursing home. "He's had some outbursts since he's been there," Zoey said. "He's had full staff called; he's injured staff. It's so awful and sad. I just wish him peace." To help Clive feel more at home, Zoey decorated his room with family photos. She loves using the pictures to tell the caregivers about Clive. She wants them to know him the way he used to be. "This is all about Clive," she said. "This is who he is; this is what his life was about. I love looking at them."

Zoey knew Clive's move away from home would be challenging for her and the kids, so she arranged for family and friends to stay at the house as a distraction. Her sister stayed the first week, her mom stayed the next week, and her best friend stayed the next. The house is significantly quieter now that Clive and his round-the-clock caregivers are no longer there.

Zoey focuses more on her own health and wellbeing now, something she hasn't done in years. "My whole life has been about Clive and Huntington's, and that's all gone suddenly," she said. "So, I've been having counseling. It's like grieving slowly. I've had times when I've felt that he has so much anger towards me. I just thought, 'I can't cope anymore; I want this to end.' I had that for ages – resenting it all – and now he's gone into a nursing home. It's like a whole other loss. It's so complex, isn't it? And there'll be another loss when he's passed. It's just so sad."

A parent's perspective

I don't fully understand how much my brother's diagnosis affected my mom. When we first learned about Huntington's disease, I was overwhelmed by my own at-risk status and concern for my brother and my at-risk family members. I think my mom and I talked about how my brother's diagnosis affected everyone but her. I knew she was worried about her affected kids and grandkids, but I will never know just how deeply that must have shaken her. Having one family member with Huntington's disease is heartbreaking enough, but potentially 10 kids and grandkids? That's the possibility my mom faced.

My mom once told me she would not have had kids if she had known Huntington's disease was in my dad's family. If that were the case, I wouldn't be here today. Perhaps that is all I need to know to understand how much learning we are an HD family affected my mom. She would rather have chosen a life without us than to have chosen a life in which she had to risk us having this disease. That's an incredibly strong statement from my very private mom who loved us dearly.

As far as being a parent to my own at-risk kids, I tried not to think about the possibility that they might have inherited Huntington's disease. The fact that they might have the expanded gene because of me made me feel at fault for something I had no control over and couldn't undo. While I remember telling my kids about my brother's diagnosis and that the three of us were at risk, most of that conversation is a blur in my memory. I do recall thinking a lot about how to tell them without paralyzing them. They took the news in stride. Like their dad, they felt that I wasn't showing symptoms, so we were all okay. I was the one who worried.

Learning that my kids and I were at risk for Huntington's disease made me think a lot about how we spent time together. My boys were teenagers when my brother was diagnosed, and my oldest was just two years away from starting college. Like other parents of high schoolers, I was mindful that the days I had with my kids at home were winding down, but learning we are an HD family made me hyper-aware. I paid more attention than I would have otherwise.

My kids were busy with their own lives, so I made a point of finding small bits of time to be around them. When they had friends over, I loved hearing the hubbub of teenage voices and laughter. I often asked my boys to tell me three interesting things about their day – an exercise they hate to this day – just to know what they found noteworthy in their lives. I wanted to take in every normal mundane moment in case there might come a day when that was no longer possible – a day when I, and maybe even they, might have Huntington's disease.

I know my HD experience would be different if I had tested positive. When I was still at risk, there was a real possibility I would develop Huntington's disease but testing negative meant that the gene-positive version of my future will never be my reality. My story diverged and took a different path the day I received my negative result. HD families with a symptomatic parent face much bigger issues than we did.

Parents in those families must determine the best way to tell their kids about Huntington's disease and help them cope with being at risk while witnessing their symptomatic parent's noticeable decline. They have countless concerns about their at-risk children's futures, as well as how they themselves will cope if one or more of their children is diagnosed with Huntington's disease. Lindsay bravely shared some of these worries throughout our conversation. Members of the HD community will be familiar with her concerns, but please reach out to a friend, family member, therapist, HD organization, or other source of support if needed.

When I spoke with Lindsay, she and her two boys – ages five and seven – were at home in Minnesota. Every now and then, one of the boys would pop into the Zoom screen, and the family dog could sometimes be heard in the background, all indications of a busy household. When Lindsay met her ex-husband, Isaac, they didn't know anything about Huntington's disease. They were pregnant with their second child when Isaac's dad was diagnosed. Instead of being concerned, they focused on the pregnancy. Lindsay thinks Isaac may have had HD symptoms as early as her first pregnancy – before his dad's diagnosis – but it took several years to recognize Isaac was showing early signs of the disease.

While Isaac's dad's most notable symptom was chorea, Isaac had more cognitive symptoms. As Lindsay said, "It presented so differently. We just didn't put it together." Looking back, though, Lindsay knows Isaac had classic HD symptoms. His work performance declined, he experienced personality changes along with depression and anxiety, he no longer made facial expressions that indicated his emotions, and he didn't seem to find joy in his two young children. Therapists and psychiatrists were unable to pinpoint what was wrong. Eventually, Lindsay filed for divorce because Isaac no longer took an active role in their relationship – or in life for that matter. When Isaac received his HD diagnosis six months later, things started to make sense. He was at least 20 years younger than his dad had been at symptom onset.

Since his diagnosis, Isaac's chorea has become more pronounced, and his cognitive ability has continued to decline. As far as Lindsay can tell, Isaac has few memories. "He seems pleasantly confused," she said. "He doesn't seem aware of the deficits, which is good. I would rather he let us worry about making decisions." Isaac lives alone now and has a simple job that gives him a small paycheck. Lindsay has power of attorney for Isaac and helps him with medical issues. "I stay involved in his care," she said. "I'm so grateful that he trusts me. His sister and I are basically the only people in his life." Two of Isaac's other siblings are gene positive, and his mom died several years ago.

Cultivating a good relationship between Isaac and their boys is very important to Lindsay, even though it takes a lot of effort. "No one will replace their dad," she said, "but I've tried to build them a family that is supportive. No one in the boys' lives speaks poorly of their dad." When the boys visit their dad's house, Lindsay's family tells the boys to be on their best behavior and help their dad out. Lindsay wants her boys to always feel like they can talk about their dad or call him when they want to. The boys spend one night every other weekend at their dad's condo. Isaac's sister often joins them, but she cannot be there all the time. Lindsay continues to assess whether it's safe for the boys to stay with their dad.

Lindsay wishes she knew more about the trajectory of Isaac's disease and how much time he has left. Lindsay is remarried, and her boys have already noticed differences between their dad and their stepdad, Dave. "Now they're in school and starting to have playdates," Lindsay said. "They see other kids and their dads, and they ask, 'Why is Daddy Dave different than Daddy Isaac? Why doesn't Dad take us places or drive or anything?' They're starting to figure that out." Lindsay worries about her boys seeing their dad's ongoing decline. When she picks them up at their dad's house, they sometimes tell her they don't want to leave. "I imagine the time that I have to tell them that they're never coming back," she said. "It's no one's fault, but it makes me so angry. Why do I have to do this? And one day, I'm going to have to tell them that he's gone and watch their little hearts break. It makes me sad."

She also worries about the day her boys learn they're at risk. Her older son already knows a little about the disease. "We talk about Huntington's. He's a smart kid, and he knows Grandpa has it, Daddy has it," Lindsay said. "At what point is he going to ask? I'm just waiting for the day, and I have no idea what I'm going to say. I would like to be prepared for when that happens." Lindsay also worries that if her boys do have Huntington's disease, they will miss out on things like having a family of their own.

Lindsay purposefully compartmentalizes the difficult parts of Huntington's disease. For her, it's easier to focus on Isaac's current needs than to think about her boys' futures. Still, she's learning to live with the uncertainty of the disease. "I'm a planner, and I want to know what is going to happen," she said. "So, not knowing? It reminds me to be present as much as I can and not worry about things that we don't have any control over. Worrying takes away the time that we have right now."

For Lindsay, the hardest thing about belonging to an HD family is contemplating whether her boys carry the expanded gene. "I can't say, well, at least one of them doesn't have it, you know? It's just the worst feeling," she said. "My life would be over." Lindsay went on to talk about her second husband and their blended family. Dave also has two kids from a previous marriage. They considered having a baby together, a child that would not be at risk for Huntington's disease. Lindsay gave it a lot of thought and finally decided she couldn't have another baby. If she loses one or both of her boys to Huntington's disease, she expects it will be too much to bear. "If both boys have it, I don't think I will want to live when they are gone," she said. "I don't want to have another baby that I would have to stay for."

Many parents of at-risk children have worries that are just as intense as Lindsay's. This concern is persistent. Not a day goes by without thoughts about whether children inherited the disease. Parents face decades of worry because children are not eligible for genetic testing until they are an adult unless their family history of Huntington's disease is accompanied by symptoms that cannot be explained by another condition. In the meantime, parents may find themselves watching their children for HD symptoms they hope will never appear. Waiting is hard, as is focusing on the present, and yet, there is nothing else to do.

A child's perspective

If my family had known about Huntington's disease, I would have had a different childhood. Without this knowledge, my parents did not have to explain to me that my dad had a degenerative brain disease that I might have inherited. Instead of lessening my burden, though, not knowing about Huntington's disease added confusion. My dad's symptoms didn't make sense, and treatment didn't seem to help. It was easy to feel annoyed or frustrated when he seemed stuck on an idea, or to feel disconnected when it was hard to carry on a conversation.

Knowing about Huntington's disease would have helped me better understand my dad, and I would have had more compassion for him. I didn't need to know about Huntington's disease to know something about my family wasn't quite right and that I could potentially have the same thing as my dad one day. I sensed that on my own. I was not protected from Huntington's disease by not knowing about it. I just experienced it in a different way.

My own childhood experiences are similar to what I see in research about HD families. Things that seemed out of the ordinary when I compared myself to my young peers seem ordinary when compared to others who grew up in HD families. When reflecting on their childhood, many people from HD families note that their HD parent's behavioral and cognitive symptoms were typically harder to cope with than the physical ones. As children, they didn't know what to expect from their HD parent, and they were often scared. Some felt like they had inadequate support or had to take care of themselves. They witnessed their HD parent's functional losses and experienced stress related to being at risk for a disease with no cure. Many experienced trauma related to being alone with an HD parent when they had sudden outbursts, choking episodes, or other distressing events. These childhood experiences affected their mental and physical health, but such impacts were reduced if they had supportive relationships with family members.

The degree to which children in HD families experience adverse situations depends on the type and severity of their parent's HD symptoms and how old a child is when their parent's symptoms begin. Some children experience adverse events throughout the course of their childhood, while others may not experience adverse events until adolescence or even adulthood. Home life typically becomes more difficult over time as a parent's symptoms progress. This was true in my family. I can recall a few uncharacteristic occurrences during my elementary school years, like my dad having outbursts over minor things. My dad's HD symptoms became established during my teenage years, when he became difficult to relate to and started having mild cognitive and behavioral symptoms. Significant events occurred as I entered young adulthood, when my dad lost his job and had two extended stays in the behavioral health unit.

When an HD parent has an earlier age of onset, children may be under a tremendous amount of stress throughout their childhood. This was Anne Elizabeth's experience. Anne Elizabeth Saldarriaga Vélez Magnusson grew up in Sweden where her father was born and raised. When we spoke, Anne Elizabeth was attending a university in her mother's home country of Colombia. Anne Elizabeth is the only remaining person in her family who might carry the expanded HD gene, and she is determined to be the last – a common hope among those in the HD community. She speaks publicly about her experiences, and she is a member of the HDYO Ambassador Executive Committee, the European Huntington Association, and the Huntington's Disease Community Advisory Board (HD-CAB).

Anne Elizabeth's early memories of her dad are of a warmhearted father who doted on her. He loved to play, and he had wanted a lot of children – enough for a full football team – but Anne Elizabeth is an only child. She was just eight years old when her dad was diagnosed with Huntington's disease. Her family talked openly about his diagnosis with family and friends, but no one told Anne Elizabeth until four years later. Her dad's neurologist thought Anne Elizabeth was too young to understand. She knows her parents were trying to protect her by following the doctor's advice, but not knowing why her dad was changing so much affected her mental health. When describing her dad, Anne Elizabeth said, "He was a great father. He was very caring, loving, patient. All of that changed drastically. He started showing psychological symptoms first – he started having paranoia, depression, anxiety. He started gaining a lot of weight. For me, it was obvious that something was going on, but nobody told me anything."

Anne Elizabeth recalls the moment she realized something had changed. Her dad screamed at her and hit her for doing something very minor that any little kid might do. "That was not my dad," she said. "When you're a kid, you blame yourself. You think it's your fault." Anne Elizabeth became very aware of her dad's moods and tried to do everything perfectly so he wouldn't have a reason to become angry. "I wish someone could have given me an instruction book – at least the basic stuff of what to do when they have outbursts." There was little information available at that time to help kids cope with the disease.

Her mom worked long hours to make sure they always had food on the table and a roof over their heads, so Anne Elizabeth was frequently home alone with her dad. "At age eight," she said, "I decided to be my father's caregiver, because I knew him the best." Even at this young age, Anne Elizabeth did the family's grocery shopping at a nearby store, kept the house spotless, and learned to make food for herself. Once she learned her dad had Huntington's disease, she felt the additional stress of knowing he was going to die someday. "Even if I take care of him – even if I do everything that I can to make sure he's okay – he'll still deteriorate and pass away," she said. "And that's such a rough reality because you don't want that for anyone."

Anne Elizabeth was frustrated when people couldn't see how bad her dad's symptoms were. He would seem fine when he was at an appointment with his neurologist or when a social worker visited. The police were called to the house several times. "Every time they came, everything looked normal," she said. "There weren't any vodka bottles anywhere, so they were like, 'It looks fine.' And since I didn't have bruises – because he only hit me three times – there wasn't something physically visible. They would say, 'No, nothing's going on. You're exaggerating.'" Even after the Swedish Huntington Association helped Anne Elizabeth document some of the things happening at home, social workers and police still didn't realize her family needed help.

Coping with a volatile father with an illness she didn't understand had a negative effect on Anne Elizabeth's mental health. She struggled to keep up with school while providing care for her dad, and she also faced a lack of understanding from friends and family. The continual stress led to anxiety, stomach pain, and possibly her obsessive-compulsive disorder. "It took a toll on me," she said. "And sadly, I tried to commit suicide because of it." After Anne Elizabeth's third suicide attempt at age 16 or 17, her dad became more involved in her life, and they developed a more positive relationship.

If Anne Elizabeth had known about Huntington's disease when her dad started showing symptoms, she thinks she would have had higher self-esteem and been able to stand up for herself. She's noticed that the message to kids today is that they are not responsible for caring for their HD parent. "They have to be kids; they have to be educated about the disease," she said. "You can't let the child care for the parent. I wish someone had told me that – told my parents that – because I shouldn't have taken that responsibility. That was too much pressure."

Anne Elizabeth's dad lived in three different care homes after he entered the late stage of Huntington's disease. He was sometimes moved without family input, and sometimes on short notice. Once, he was moved to a care home that was two and a half hours away and not easily accessible by bus. This made it challenging for Anne Elizabeth to visit because she didn't have a driver's license. When her dad was moved to a care home specifically for HD patients, he was much happier. He liked that his chorea didn't set him apart from others, and he made several friends. When Anne Elizabeth was no longer her dad's caregiver, they were able to have genuine father-daughter time. Her dad especially liked playing a bowling video game. Despite his chorea, he almost always won.

When Anne Elizabeth sought out genetic testing at age 18, she was told it would be better to wait until after college because it could be hard to cope with a test result while working on her degree and caring for her dad. Soon after she finished her degree, Anne Elizabeth moved to Colombia and then the COVID-19 pandemic began. It still wasn't a good time to get tested. So, for now, she goes to the HD clinic every year for a battery of behavioral, cognitive, and motor tests to determine if she has any early symptoms of the disease. She passes every year, which eases her anxiety and insomnia.

She expects she'll get tested when the time feels right whether that's after finishing her next degree or if she has a future partner who's interested in having kids. Anne Elizabeth is not scared of having Huntington's disease, and she values the time she has now to live a full life. "I want to use my healthy, young years doing everything that I can," she said. "It's better to enjoy life. I might test negative, and then I can say I did all this stuff, and now I can do even more."

While Anne Elizabeth has gone to counseling most of her life, not every therapist has known about Huntington's disease or how it affects young people who are at risk. She now sees a psychologist in Colombia who has worked wonders. "I haven't been this happy in a while," she said. In addition, Anne Elizabeth continues to feel supported by the Swedish Huntington Association, especially the director who knows a lot about Huntington's disease and is easy to talk to. Anne Elizabeth can say anything, and the director understands. "She is like my second mom – always making sure I'm okay."

Before Anne Elizabeth left Sweden, she knew her dad was very sick and might pass away soon. She spent six hours with him on their last visit. "I told him I was going to miss him a lot and I loved him a lot – giving hugs and making sure that he wouldn't feel left behind," she said. A few months later, her dad became gravely ill with pneumonia. Anne Elizabeth was half a world away, but a nurse helped her get a recorded video message to him. In it, Anne Elizabeth told her dad how much she loved him, and she included one of his favorite songs. The hospital called 12 minutes after playing the video to tell her he had died.

As Anne Elizabeth talked about her dad's death, she likened it to a circle in her life. When Anne Elizabeth was born, her mom had serious childbirth complications, so her dad was the first person to welcome her into this world. He was very happy to have her in his life. Before her dad died, Anne Elizabeth connected with him through her video message from the other side of the world. She was the last one to be with him, and she was very happy to have had him in her life. "It's sad, but it's happy at the same time because the final person he heard was me," she said. "I was happy about that in the end. It was beautiful to close that circle." Given the choice, Anne Elizabeth doesn't think she would pick a different life.

A family disease ties family members together in a unique way. As a member of an HD family, I don't just think about tracing my family tree or pinpointing the places my family has called home. I don't just think about whether I inherited my mom's eye color or my dad's sense of organization. Instead, Huntington's disease has inserted a more pervasive link to my family's past, as well as our future. We are linked by the shared experience of a devastating family disease – a family disease with a pattern of loss that is repeating across generations of my family.

Huntington's disease connects me and my family members across time. It's like a web that reaches back in time to parents, aunts, uncles, and grandparents; across the present to siblings and cousins; and forward in time to children, nieces, nephews, and grandchildren. Its reach is extensive and persistent. I feel strong ties to my family's HD roots, and even though I don't have the disease, it continues to have power over me. It affects my identity, my mental and emotional wellbeing, and my relationships with family members. My family's genetic history is as much a part of who I am as my childhood memories or my grandma's family stories.

CHILDREN WITH HUNTINGTON'S DISEASE

Before I tested negative for Huntington's disease, I tried not to think about the possibility that my boys might have the disease one day. It was surreal to know their HD gene status had already been decided, and there was nothing I could do to change it. Thinking about my boys having the disease as adults was hard enough, but if I had noticed symptoms when they were still children? That would have been another story. Huntington's disease is a cruel disease in adults, and it is even more severe when it strikes children. It would have been excruciating to watch my kids decline at such a young age.

Juvenile Huntington's disease (JHD) is a particularly devastating form of the disease in which HD symptoms appear before the age of 20. Most, but not all, cases of Juvenile Huntington's disease are inherited from a father. Children with Juvenile Huntington's disease have very long CAG repeats – often 60 repeats or more – that are typically associated with an earlier age of onset, faster progression, and more severe disease. In one extreme example, researchers documented the case of a boy with a CAG repeat greater than 200 who developed symptoms before the age of two. Some children have symptoms at the same time as their HD parent, and some even develop symptoms before their parent does.

In both the juvenile and adult forms of Huntington's disease, physical and cognitive decline are combined with behavioral changes, and symptoms and disease progression vary widely from person to person. There are some distinct differences, however. Compared to the adult form, Juvenile Huntington's disease causes more atrophy in certain areas of the brain. It has some unique potential symptoms as well, including seizures, poor muscle control, abnormal muscle tightness, and itching. The older a child is when symptoms appear, the more their symptoms look like adult-onset Huntington's disease. Chorea is uncommon in Juvenile Huntington's disease unless symptom onset is in the later teen years.

While almost all cases of Juvenile Huntington's disease have a known family history, its early arrival is often a surprise. Huntington's disease typically manifests in adulthood, and Juvenile Huntington's disease is very rare, so parents may be caught off guard when they see significant changes in their child. If a child is adopted or their HD parent is no longer part of their life, Juvenile Huntington's disease may not even be on anyone's radar. A child exhibiting early JHD symptoms may have trouble paying attention, or they may develop new learning difficulties. They may have changes in behavior or show signs of depression, aggression, or suicidal ideation. They might also have difficulty controlling natural urges that appear during puberty. Most notably, they become markedly different from the child they once were.

Rarest of the rare

Juvenile Huntington's disease makes up only five to ten percent of all cases of Huntington's disease and is estimated to affect fewer than 5,000 young people in the United States. Having a rare form of a rare disease compounds the challenges associated with Huntington's disease. General practitioners know even less about Juvenile Huntington's disease than they do about Huntington's disease, and doctors specializing in Juvenile Huntington's disease are few and far between. JHD families have fewer resources to help them understand and cope with the disease. When Juvenile Huntington's disease is mentioned in HD resources, it is sometimes relegated to a small space, almost like an afterthought.

Research shows that parents of children with any rare disease face multiple challenges. They are often dissatisfied with how much medical professionals know about their child's disease. Their finances and ability to work are often impaired by needing to provide care for their child, and they feel isolated and alone in facing their child's rare disease. Social interactions are affected, and it becomes difficult to maintain friendships. To cope, many parents compartmentalize and suppress complicated feelings, while others do their best to focus on the present. These findings were reflected in many of my conversations, not just those with JHD parents.

Parents in JHD families watch their child decline as other children around them thrive. Their child's world becomes smaller at a time of life when other children can look ahead to limitless possibilities. Parents do their best to give their child the best life possible in a short amount of time. That was the case for Bill and Karen, who were at home in Tennessee when we spoke. Bill is a physician, and Karen is a nurse. Their adopted son, Brian, had died of Juvenile Huntington's disease when he was 31 years old.

Over the years, Bill and Karen met only a small number of JHD families, and they found few JHD resources, especially resources specifically for young people who have Juvenile Huntington's disease. Most youth and young adults in HD families need support because they have a parent with Huntington's disease, they're considering genetic testing, or they're coping with their at-risk or gene-positive status. Very few youth in the HD community are also coping with JHD's debilitating symptoms. "There's not a support group for young people with progressive dementia," Bill said. "You're kind of alone for that."

At the beginning of our conversation, Bill and Karen were eager to show me a picture of Brian as a young adult – when he could still walk and talk. It was of utmost importance to give Brian a face – to make him real to me – before they delved into the details of their family's JHD journey. They knew Brian was at risk for Huntington's disease when they adopted him, but they didn't discuss it with him when he was young. They didn't know anyone with Huntington's disease, so there was no natural opportunity for Brian to ask questions or for Bill and Karen to explain the disease little by little over the years.

Bill and Karen were hopeful Brian had not inherited the expanded gene, so it didn't make sense to worry about something Brian might not have to face. Besides, if Brian had inherited Huntington's disease, Bill and Karen expected it would be decades before symptoms appeared. In hindsight, Bill wonders if they should have shared more with Brian once it became clear he was having cognitive and behavioral changes. At the time, however, giving this news to a teenaged son who was already struggling didn't seem wise.

Brian's first symptoms appeared around age 10 when school assignments that had once been manageable became too challenging. After several years of struggling in the public school system, Brian attended private school, and then Bill and Karen homeschooled him for the last two years of high school. Homeschooling allowed them to incorporate activities like concerts, plays, ski trips, and roller coasters, into Brian's education – experiences he wouldn't have had if he was in a traditional school setting.

Bill and Karen chuckled often as they talked about Brian's "adventures," even when the events they described were far from humorous at the time. Brian's impulsivity got him into many predicaments. He had multiple interactions with the police, went to juvenile court several times, and totaled his car and lost his license at age 16. When Brian wanted to enlist in the US Air Force, he passed the rigorous physical and mental tests despite having HD-related coordination and cognitive issues. Bill and Karen worried he wouldn't do well in the service and encouraged him to get tested for Huntington's disease before committing. When Brian's test result came back with a

CAG repeat of 58, he did not enlist. After Brian tested positive, Bill and Karen facilitated classes with the police department to teach officers about Huntington's disease and help them understand what Brian and others in the HD community faced.

When Brian was a young adult, he disappeared for days at a time. "He lived in a different world," Bill said. "One time, he slept in the forest because he thought guys were chasing him for money." Karen continued, "We bought him snow pants and a jacket because he was sleeping on railroad tracks. We'd find him and get him cleaned up and showered, and he'd go back out with his friends. He was always hiding from somebody." After an unsuccessful attempt at culinary school, Brian had trouble maintaining a job and his apartment. Bill and Karen noticed several people coming and going from Brian's life, and sometimes Brian's belongings disappeared with them. He moved back home at the age of 19 and lost the ability to work altogether soon after.

One day, Brian told his parents he was going to take a nap. It wasn't long before the police and a crisis counselor knocked on their door. Unbeknownst to Bill and Karen, Brian had told a friend he was going to kill himself. While Brian did not seriously harm himself, Bill thinks this episode was just one indication of how difficult it was for Brian to face his diagnosis. "He had self-injurious behavior," Bill said. "He would burn himself with a cigarette, and he was pretty depressed. We tried working with a neurologist. Life was stolen from him. He was angry. He would rip up the Bible if we talked to him about HD. 'What god would do this?' he would say. It was very hard for him – very hard for us."

Caring for Brian was extremely stressful. "He smoked and got to the point where he couldn't light his own cigarettes, so he would ask us to light them," Bill said. "He would sleep for 48 hours at a time and be awake for 48 hours at a time. We were both working, and we worried about him burning the house down – worried about him hurting himself. We tag-teamed caring for him, and for a while we hired help during the day." Figuring out sleep medication for Brian changed their lives for the better.

Karen talked about two chapters of Brian's disease. The first chapter was dominated by Brian's behavioral symptoms, which she described as, "impulsive, angry, disappearing, sometimes violent, arguing…" Bill interjected to say, "It was a continuous horrible." The second chapter started when Brian became completely dependent on others for all activities of daily living, such as dressing, showering, toileting, and eating. "When he couldn't walk, couldn't talk, it was also terrible," Karen said, "but we didn't have those behavioral episodes anymore."

One particularly difficult aspect of Juvenile Huntington's disease is meeting a child's end-of-life needs, which often requires 24-hour skilled nursing care. Most long-term care facilities have little or no experience meeting the unique needs of a child or young person with Juvenile Huntington's disease. In the United States, some states do not even have nursing home beds for people younger than 16.

Bill and Karen chose to care for Brian at home rather than move him to a care facility. They knew they had the skills to care for him, and they hired caregivers to help. Most importantly, Brian was happy at home. Bill and Karen made modifications to their house to accommodate Brian's needs. He had a hospital bed, a ceiling-mounted lift and harness to move him, and a renovated bathroom. His bedroom had large windows with a nice view. "He spent a lot of time here," Karen said. "He had a big TV. We'd come in every night and sit with him after he got his medications. He'd settle down and get sleepy."

When Brian was alive, it was hard for Bill to find hope in their situation. "It was kind of a hopeless situation in my mind," Bill said. "The only hope was the development of a treatment, and it was pretty obvious that that was going to be at a snail's pace and the disease at a rapid pace. Unfortunately, Brian was not going to benefit. Our hope was to make him happy and comfortable. If I could get him to smile, that would be great. Later, if we could get him to eat, that would be great. Keep him comfortable and not have anything bad happen, you know? We tried to make his life as happy as could be and make this the best-equipped spa that we could have for as short of a life as he had."

Brian died right before the COVID-19 pandemic began. Even though Juvenile Huntington's disease is no longer part of their everyday lives,

Bill and Karen continue to advocate for the HD community. Early in their JHD journey, Bill and Karen looked for ways to fill gaps in what was available to help HD families, and especially JHD families. HDSA has many Centers of Excellence that provide clinical care and services to HD families throughout the United States. When Brian was first diagnosed, there was no Center of Excellence in the area, so Bill worked with the head of neurology at Vanderbilt Hospital to start one. Bill and Karen are members of HD-CAB and continue to serve the HD community even though they no longer have a family member with the disease.

Shining light on a rare disease

Parents of children with Juvenile Huntington's disease often sense that something isn't quite right with their child long before they seek a diagnosis, and some feel like they know their child has Juvenile Huntington's disease before their suspicion is confirmed. It can be challenging, however, to reach a JHD diagnosis. Very few doctors have expertise in Juvenile Huntington's disease. Most general practitioners have never had a JHD patient, so they may be unfamiliar with its symptoms. Even within HDSA's system of Centers of Excellence, only some centers have doctors specializing in the juvenile form of the disease. To work with a JHD expert, many families must travel to another state, which can be difficult due to the financial burden and stresses related to travel.

Genetic testing protocols developed by HDSA recommend not testing children under the age of 18 unless there is a medical reason to do so, such as receiving a clinical diagnosis from a neurologist. Other conditions must be ruled out first. This is true even if there is a known family history of Huntington's disease. There are many childhood conditions with symptoms in common with Huntington's disease, so it can be challenging to determine if a child's symptoms are caused by

Juvenile Huntington's disease, normal developmental changes, or another condition like autism, attention-deficit/hyperactivity disorder (ADHD), or a learning disability. Additionally, the stress of living in an HD household can cause anxiety, disrupted sleep, acting out, and other behaviors that could be misinterpreted as early signs of the disease. Even though these symptoms cause families a lot of worry, symptom management is the same with or without a JHD diagnosis.

While parents may want to know their child's HD gene status, HDSA testing protocols do not consider this enough of a reason for a child to undergo genetic testing. There are reasons for being cautious and taking time. Ruling out other diagnoses can take several years, and there are major implications if a child is tested too soon. A child with Juvenile Huntington's disease typically has a CAG repeat larger than 60, but a child could be tested and receive a positive result in the typical adult-onset range of 40 to 50 CAG repeats. In this case, the child would learn at a young age that they will develop Huntington's disease as an adult, but the result would not explain their current symptoms. The child would also lose the ability to make the genetic testing decision for themselves when they turn 18. A child living in a stressful home environment in which a parent is exhibiting HD symptoms could be particularly devastated by knowing they will develop Huntington's disease when they grow up.

Parents of children with Juvenile Huntington's disease must cope with helping their child face a devastating family disease – something families may do with little support, few resources, and little understanding from others. But some JHD families, like Londen Tabor and her daughter, Autumn, are trying to change this by using social media to raise awareness and advocate for JHD families. When I spoke with Londen, she was at home in Wyoming, and Autumn was about to turn 17.

Londen's journey with Huntington's disease began when she met Autumn's dad, Justin, when they were both just 19 years old. Justin told Londen early in their relationship that his mom died of Huntington's disease when he was in the third grade, and it was possible he could have the disease when he got older. Londen had never heard of it, so she didn't think it was a big deal. Now, though, she recalls Justin already had neck tics and other slight symptoms when they met. Londen became very concerned several years later when more symptoms appeared.

Londen and Justin were together for six years and had two children – Autumn and her brother – but they never married before they broke up. Justin adored his kids and thought of Londen's older son from a previous relationship as one of his own. As Londen said, "His kids were his life." Justin tested positive soon after their breakup, so Londen thinks his HD symptoms likely played a role in many of their arguments. When Justin eventually needed long-term care, he moved to a nursing home close to Londen. He was by far the youngest resident there. The kids loved spending time with their dad. They would ride their bikes down the street to visit him, and they sometimes spent the night in his room on cots. They invited their dad to school events and showed no embarrassment when other kids stared at him.

When Londen met her husband, Chris, she was unsure about bringing a new person into her life. She was cautious about getting too involved. "I got scared," she said. "I didn't want to get myself in too deep because there was no way he was going to take care of my children the way I'd need him to. Who would want to do that?" She was wrong, though. When Londen and Chris got engaged, the kids couldn't wait to tell their dad. Londen was hesitant to share the news, but Justin's excitement was apparent when he asked to see the ring with a big grin on his face. Since then, Chris has been by Londen's side. "Chris is my rock," she said. "He has literally supported me and held my hand and helped guide me through all of this. If I didn't have him, I wouldn't be here. I found the love of my life. I really did."

Londen's at-risk children started participating in the Kids-HD study at the University of Iowa's HDSA Center of Excellence when Autumn was six years old. Kids-HD is a brain imaging study that focuses on young people from HD families; it has since been renamed ChANGE-HD. Autumn and her at-risk brother visit the university annually to have an MRI and complete a series of cognitive and physical assessments. "I'm so glad we started when we did," Londen said, "because the data they have on Autumn – from her not having any manifestations of the disease in 2012 to seeing that progression in brain scans – that's so important for research."

Autumn started having significant behavioral changes around the time she turned 10. At first, Londen thought Autumn might be entering puberty, but it gradually became clear that something else was going on. Autumn had been diagnosed with ADHD, but this looked different. "I remember crying because Autumn was having these crazy fits and going nuts over nothing," Londen said. "It was not like her. It was weird and scary." This was a complete change from how Londen described Autumn before her symptoms appeared. "Autumn was always laughing and giggling and singing songs and sassing. She liked to make people laugh. I think because of her dad, she's always wanted to help people. That little girl – she's still in there; it's just harder to come out."

As Autumn's symptoms progressed, it became harder to dismiss the possibility that she might have Juvenile Huntington's disease, so Autumn met with a pediatric neurologist the next time she was at the University of Iowa. The doctor had some concerns, but the first step was to rule out other potential explanations. Over the next few months, however, Autumn continued to change. She began getting in trouble at school, and slight physical movements appeared. "To get her the proper help, I needed a proper diagnosis," Londen said. "And hey, if it wasn't JHD, then that would have been even better." The doctors at University of Iowa agreed it was time to bring Autumn back to Iowa to get tested. Her genetic test result was positive.

When Autumn received her positive result, the first thing she wanted to do was tell her dad. "She wanted him to know that he wasn't alone – that she had it, too," Londen said. Justin's biggest fear had always been that his kids would have Huntington's disease. Londen cried as she recounted her visit with Justin later that day. He was in the last stage of Huntington's disease and no longer able to speak. "Tears were streaming down his face," she said. "He and I just sat there, and we cried together."

Londen used to tell Justin stupid jokes to get him to smile, especially after he was no longer able to talk. "That smile always made me know that he was still there," Londen said as she cried. "And the last week before he died, I couldn't get him to smile. That's how I knew it was towards the end." Londen and the kids spent the night in Justin's room the night he died, and Londen held his hand as he passed away at the age of 36, just six months after Autumn's diagnosis.

Having a child with Juvenile Huntington's disease draws much of the family's attention away from siblings who are at risk or gene negative. "For the longest time, people thought Autumn was my only kid. It's not surprising," Londen said. Her sons are both old enough to live away from home. "They know what it means for their little sister to have JHD because they saw how the disease affected their dad. The boys are loving and supportive of their sister, but they don't ever talk to me about their sadness. I know it hurts them to see how she's declined." So far, Londen's at-risk son shows no sign of the disease. "There are no symptoms, so he doesn't feel the need to get tested," Londen said. "For him – unless he's planning to have kids – there isn't a reason. He thinks he's fine. I agree. All I can do is have hope he doesn't have it."

Chris adopted Autumn after Justin died, but by then, the boys were too old. Preparing for what lies ahead for their family is hard to think about, and Londen and Chris often don't make decisions before they have to. For example, Autumn is having difficulty controlling her muscles to clear her throat, so she chokes a lot, but Londen and Chris are not hurrying into the decision to insert a feeding tube. "We'll put it off until we have to deal with it," Londen said. "And it's probably not good because you want to prepare for things, but at the same time, it's so painful. The only way for me to get through each day is to not think about the future. I know what's going to happen. I know children who have passed away from JHD. How am I going to handle that? It's so scary."

One way Londen copes with Autumn's disease is to keep her mind focused on things unrelated to Juvenile Huntington's disease. "I could tell you everything you want to know about the Oregon Trail," she said. Londen recently stopped drinking alcohol, something she had relied on to cope with depression, and she started learning jujitsu, a sport her husband loves. She also focuses her attention on advocacy and raising awareness.

Londen is passionate about making it possible for kids with Juvenile Huntington's disease to participate in clinical trials. Since there is no treatment or cure, participating in clinical trials would offer some hope. Currently, though, children with Juvenile Huntington's disease are not eligible to participate until they turn 18, by which time many have symptoms that have progressed too far to benefit from any potential treatment. Other children pass away before their 18th birthday. "Clinical trials are coming fast," Londen said. "And before you know it, there will be a treatment. It breaks my heart to know that for my daughter, I feel like there is no hope. I wish I had a tiny bit of hope, but as much as I want to put myself in that positive mindset, I worry about false hope. So instead, I just hope for the best. That's all I can do."

Londen recently joined six other JHD parents to meet with a panel from the US Food and Drug Administration (FDA) to make a case for allowing minors with Juvenile Huntington's disease to participate in clinical trials. When it was Londen's turn to speak, she chose not to focus on Autumn's symptoms. Instead, Londen said, "I wanted to tell a story about how much I love my daughter, and all the things I would do for my child just like they would for their children. I wanted them to see the amazing, beautiful girl that she was. In the end, our stories literally came together and told one sadly amazing story that I think was really touching to the FDA. I also wanted to make sure that the FDA knew that we were just seven families. We were lucky enough to have this opportunity, but there are so many of us out there that need this help."

The title of their FDA presentation was, "About Me: I grieve the past, I grieve the present, and I grieve the future." Londen cried as she said, "Literally, I do… I do. It hurts to look at old stuff from when your child was the person that you know is still there, but now they're gone – wondering what she'd be doing right now, which friends she'd be hanging out with, what job she would have. She'd probably be volunteering at the animal shelter." Londen's tears kept coming.

"Autumn was beautiful – she still is... She was amazing – she still is... You can just feel her vibes, you know?"

Londen used to revel in the community aspect of national HD conventions. She already knew a lot about Huntington's disease, so she attended to connect with others. When Londen went to her first convention after Autumn's diagnosis, however, she felt more alone than she ever had. "I was trying to be strong, but I felt so alone in a community that I had been a part of for years," Londen said. "I'm now here as a JHD parent, and I'm looking around, and my kid can't be in clinical trials. I had never thought about what if this happens to my kid, you know? I was very frustrated. I felt like nobody understood me. I was so broken inside, and I just wanted to find my people and my people weren't there. I felt alone. I went on the internet, and there was nothing about JHD, so I just shut down."

By the next annual convention, Autumn's symptoms were getting worse, but there was still no one talking about Juvenile Huntington's disease. Instead, there was excitement about the increasing number of clinical trials for adults and the hope that they would lead to a cure. "For clinical trials, timing is everything," Londen said. "Ten years from now, there'll probably be something that she can have, but she won't be here. I was mad that I was wasting time on all this when my daughter was literally dying. I wish that our HD community understood our JHD community more, and I wish there was more available for JHD kids like there is for adults with this disease."

Londen struggled after that convention. "This was worse than depression," she said. "I just had to tell myself that Autumn's here today. There may be things that she can't do, but we can still go out and do the things that she *can* do. We can still give her the best life possible: make her laugh; be her best friend; make up for the friends she doesn't have." After that convention, Chris drove the kids home from the airport, while Londen drove her own car. Along the way, she recorded dozens of videos expressing her sadness, anger, and frustration. She has yet to watch them, but she found the process of expressing her feelings therapeutic. It was during this drive that she decided that if no one else was going to make a change, she was going to do it herself.

She wanted to start a conversation about Juvenile Huntington's disease and get people to listen, so she decided to share not only what she and her family were going through, but also what the larger JHD community was going through. She started making YouTube videos, but they didn't gain much traction. Then, Londen discovered TikTok. It was tough to build a platform of JHD followers, so she uploaded videos about her home state of Wyoming. They went viral. Once she hit 10,000 followers, she switched it up and started talking about Juvenile Huntington's disease. She now has more than 160,000 TikTok followers.

"I've inspired other people to be like, 'I'm going through this, too.' And we've all connected, and now we do feel a sense of not being alone," she said. "The #JuvenileHuntingtionsDisease hashtag had no views on TikTok when it started, and it now has over 16 million views. #HuntingtonsDisease had like 1,000 views, and now that has like 24 million. It's amazing, and you know what? I will take credit for being the start of that. I'm proud of that, and I'm so happy when I see other people on the platform."

When posting on social media, Londen intentionally avoids mentioning the most difficult parts of Autumn's disease. "I try to make videos that are educational," she said. "I try to stay as positive as I can because that's the only way for me to get through life. Otherwise, I'll get stuck back in that hole I was in for 18 months of being angry and sad and worried and scared. And before you know it, my daughter will be gone. So, my way of coping is to continue educating, continue finding and creating resources for people, continue encouraging, continue inspiring, and continue sharing in the hope that we'll make a difference for everybody else. Yes, HD is out there, and it is a rare disease, but hello – these are our children. Our voices have been heard, and things are changing."

Londen continues to raise awareness for Juvenile Huntington's disease. In addition to being active on social media, she started her own podcast called, *The JHD Journal*. She appears on others' podcasts, speaks publicly, and thinks about writing a book someday. It might be a children's book that she writes with Autumn's input, or it might be a book about her own life. "I try not to think about it," Londen said, "but I know that in the future I will have more time on my hands, and I will need to find ways to cope, and maybe writing a book will be one of those ways."

In many ways, Juvenile Huntington's disease is a concentrated form of Huntington's disease. It strikes earlier, and it tends to progress quicker and have more intense symptoms than the adult form. Parents of children with Juvenile Huntington's disease are in a race against time – every day matters to these families. Their child's ability to walk, talk, play, and just be a kid dwindles as time passes, and these kids know it.

JHD parents don't want their kids to suffer. They want their children to have as much joy in their lives as possible, so they make tough decisions about their child's medical care, become their child's best friend, and devote their lives to their child's needs – all to create the most livable life possible for their children.

RELATING TO A LOVED ONE WITH HUNTINGTON'S DISEASE

My early childhood memories of my dad are somewhat vague but overall positive. I remember playing with him in our yard. I remember watching him shave in the mornings, sometimes while I sang songs. He instigated family day trips to explore the natural beauty around us, and he taught me how to ski and how to shake hands with a firm grip. He often told me I could be anything I wanted to be when I grew up. But he changed gradually over time and became hard to talk to, unreasonable, and easy to anger. Without knowing about Huntington's disease, I thought these traits were a true reflection of who he was.

When I learned I was at risk for Huntington's disease, one of my fears was becoming like my dad. I didn't want to become inaccessible, misunderstood, and unwell. I didn't want to become hard to relate to and interact with. I hated to think about my family developing these types of feelings about me, especially since I would need my family's support if I developed Huntington's disease one day. It was easy to worry that my ties to those I love the most might not be strong enough to withstand the challenges of Huntington's disease. What would I do if I had to face this disease all by myself? I am certain my family wouldn't completely abandon me, but I couldn't stop the doubts from creeping in. I was in a very vulnerable position.

Now that I understand why things were so difficult with my dad, I can't help wishing I could tell him I'm sorry for how I felt when I misinterpreted his HD symptoms as his true self. I also wish we had known we needed to appreciate the time we had with my dad before he started developing HD symptoms. We had no idea what was coming, so he slipped below the surface of Huntington's disease with no indication of where he was going or that he would not return

By the time I was old enough to really know my dad, he was already symptomatic. I know facts about my dad, but I didn't get to know his true personality. I only have sparse clues about what he was really like. I wish I knew how to piece them together and fill in the gaps to create a whole version of my dad uninfluenced by Huntington's disease. I continue looking for ways to connect with him because I think it's an important part of my own HD journey. My efforts to know my dad better won't change anything for him, but they mean everything to me. Getting to know my dad matters, even if I'm decades too late.

If I could go back in time, I would love to talk to my dad as a young man. I would love to know what he was like before he started having HD symptoms. I wonder what I would find familiar about him, and what would surprise me. Am I like him in any way? What would it be like to have an easy back-and-forth conversation with him, and what stories would he tell me? Would he be funny or wise? And what would he want

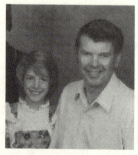

Me and my dad.

to know about me and my kids? I'm sure he would smile a lot. I'm curious about this person I will never truly know.

Connecting with an HD parent

The cognitive and behavioral symptoms of Huntington's disease plus its genetic component have a major impact on the relationship between an HD parent and their child. A child may experience their parent's outbursts, violence, suicidal ideation, or other upsetting symptoms. A child may be embarrassed to be seen in public with their parent, especially if people stare or their parent is mistaken for being drunk or on drugs. Children may be afraid to invite friends over or feel guilty for having negative thoughts about their HD parent. Alternatively, they may feel protective of their HD parent. At the same time, children face the possibility – or the certainty – of having the same disease themselves one day. The nature of this relationship affects how children in HD families view their own potential future with the disease. When I was still at risk, the way I thought about my future was heavily influenced by how I experienced my dad's disease.

In most of my conversations with the HD community, I asked, "Do you remember what your parent was like before they developed HD symptoms?" I wanted to understand how long HD symptoms had affected the parent-child relationship and whether people felt like they'd had a chance to really know their mom or dad. This question is tied to a lot of complex feelings. People's voices became animated or cracked with emotion as they shared memories from the past. Sometimes, the question induced smiles, other times tears, and often both. Some people no longer recognize their HD parent as the person they used to be due to the extent of their HD symptoms. Others were too young when their HD parent started having symptoms to remember the pre-HD version of their mom or dad. Many people shared a sense of loss related to knowing their HD parent will not be present for major life events.

Many HD families make extra effort to spend time together so children will have positive recollections of what their HD parent was like before symptom onset. Families know this time is limited. As a parent's disease progresses, it is not easy to hold on to the parent-child relationship that existed before HD symptoms appeared, nor is it easy to create and maintain a new form of that relationship when a parent is no longer able to interact as they once did. Eventually, the relationship between a child and their HD parent relies heavily on memories – some good, some bad.

In many of my conversations, it was apparent that maintaining this relationship in some form is a central part of the HD experience. I know it is part of my experience, even now. Finn is an at-risk young man from the United States who was very young when his dad became symptomatic, so he feels like he doesn't really know his dad. "I don't remember much of him otherwise," Finn said. "I can't think of a conversation we've had where it's been normal." Finn tries to find ways to connect with the father he never knew as well as the symptomatic father he knows now.

Finn sees hints of what his dad used to be like in old photos and home movies. He hopes these glimpses of his dad before symptom onset will help him get to know his dad a little better. "I found one photo where I think we kind of look alike," Finn said. "We have the same sort of smile. No one ever says we look alike, so I saved that photo." When watching old home movies of his dad, Finn finds it strange to see a person he should know but doesn't. He sees things about his dad that are no longer visible, like the way he used to move before he developed chorea. Finn recently pored over his parents' wedding album. "It was kind of fun, but it was weird at the same time," he said. "It's strange to see my dad look like a normal, functioning person – standing up and dancing. It's fun to see the person people talk about."

As the youngest child in his family, Finn witnessed some of his dad's most difficult episodes, many of which occurred after his siblings left home. While it wasn't easy for his siblings, they were able to escape to a more normal day-to-day existence at college. Finn sometimes wishes he'd also had the chance to leave before things got bad, but he's glad he's been able to support his mom. Finn is thinking of moving out now that he's done with school and has a steady job. After being there for his mom for so long, though, he worries about leaving. The two of them have faced the most challenging parts of his dad's disease together.

Finn was 13 years old when his dad became the first person in their family to receive an HD diagnosis. Finn and his siblings each coped with learning they are at risk in different ways. Finn became accustomed to constant anxiety that he deals with by going to therapy and learning as much as he can about Huntington's disease; one sibling was in denial for many years, pushing aside thoughts of Huntington's disease as much as possible; and the other sibling turned to substance abuse.

There are times when Finn can't stop thinking about Huntington's disease. "I don't want to think about it all the time. I don't like the anxiety of whether I'm positive or negative," he said. He recently realized just how much it was on his mind when a co-worker's mom had a stroke. Seeing a friend struggle with a parent's health issues brought up a lot of complex feelings and emotions for Finn. He knows how important it is to feel like those around you understand what's happening in your life, so he tries to check on people when they're having a tough time. "I had a little chat with him and tried to ask more than just how his mom was doing. I asked how he was doing and if he needed a break." Finn got a hug in return.

Finn hasn't told many people about Huntington's disease because he's unsure of how they'll react. Recently, he got tired of pretending that everything is fine – that his dad is fine – so he started talking about his dad at work. He hasn't gone so far as to mention that his dad has Huntington's disease, but some of his co-workers now know his dad uses a wheelchair, and at least one co-worker knows his dad no longer lives at home because of health issues. "I feel like no one knows me at work because they don't know this part of my life," he said. "So, yeah, it's a good thing to work on more."

Contemplating what adulthood will look like is much different now than it was before his dad's diagnosis. When Finn and his friends used to talk about getting old, he would think about what kind of grandpa he wanted to be, but now it's hard to figure out how to participate in those conversations. He also wonders how his at-risk status will affect romantic relationships. "I don't want to say it on the first date, but eventually, early on, I should let the person know these things about me," he said. "I don't want them to feel like I've tricked them." Finn also thinks about whether he wants to have kids one day. Based on his own childhood experience, he's not sure he wants to raise kids in a home with a gene-positive parent.

It's been hard for Finn to watch his dad's decline and wonder if the same thing will happen to him. "That's one of my main fears," he said. "A huge reason I want to get tested is that the idea of being in his position – where you mentally can't get out of it, and you're stuck in your body until you die – that scares me a lot. If life is going to be like what he's experiencing, I don't feel like it would be worth sticking around." Finn also worries about what it would be like to live in a long-term care setting. When he worked in a nursing home, some employees didn't treat the residents well. He thinks having a complicated disease that is often misunderstood and requires a lot of care increases the risk of being mistreated.

Finn didn't used to worry that dropping things or tripping meant he was gene positive because he felt too young to have symptoms. He didn't anticipate getting tested until his life was more settled and after gaining more world experience – probably when he was closer to age 30. He said he wanted to be, "in a clear space and as calm as possible." Now, though, Finn knows people his age who are showing symptoms. "That feels different to me," he said. "It feels like more of a possibility now, so I've had a lot of anxiety." Finn is starting to think he might get tested in the next few years so he can know what to expect in the future. "It's definitely something I think about actively." He might talk to a genetic counselor to get the perspective of someone outside his family before making that decision.

Finn's dad has lived in two different group homes in the last seven years, and each has taken a different approach to his dad's care. Finn knows it's not easy to care for someone with Huntington's disease, but he thinks staff at the first group home didn't try to find the best ways to work with his dad. "It seemed like they were having trouble, so they drugged him," Finn said. "And then he was too much for them." Finn thinks the group home could have communicated better with his family about the difficulties of caring for an HD patient. It was a missed opportunity for the staff to learn more and provide the best care.

The second group home is a much better fit. Its supportive environment has had a positive impact on his dad's mental state. A caregiver with experience in caring for an HD patient has been a huge benefit. "She pays attention to details," Finn said. "She doesn't leave snacks in his room. He has to come out to the kitchen to avoid choking. She understands he needs a lot of food because he moves constantly, and he can get really cold. Those things are HD-specific." Finn's dad seems more comfortable in the new group home, and his family feels more welcome. "It feels like they want us there to support him," Finn said.

Finn's dad's ability to communicate has declined. He still engages during family visits, but for the most part, he only answers questions with simple answers. Finn and his family have had to find new ways to relate to his dad. Finn misses the days when his dad could still call or text, and he knows his dad will continue to change. "I can't connect much with my dad at all now," he said. "When I'm alone with him, I don't know how to have a conversation, so it's hard to visit. I try to remember that he probably isn't thinking it's awkward at all, even if it's silent."

Finn often wonders what his dad would be like now if he didn't have Huntington's disease. Would he be proud of Finn and what he's accomplished? What kinds of questions would he ask about Finn's life? During a recent visit, Finn noted that his dad never said anything the entire time. "I'm definitely an introvert," Finn said, "so trying to talk about myself for a half hour is difficult." Talking about family memories or favorite bands has been one way to get responses from his dad, and Finn recognizes his dad's sense of humor when he laughs at funny comments. Finn remembers hating his dad's Dad Jokes when he was in middle school. "Every night at dinner, he would say, 'You know Finn, one day you're going to realize just how funny I am.' And now I know how funny he is. It took a while to see it, but now I know."

Relationships change as symptoms progress

HD symptoms can make a loved one challenging to live with, and it can be hard to separate a person from their disease. Conflicts can arise when declining abilities prevent a loved one with Huntington's disease from meeting others' expectations of what they can or should be able to do. A person with Huntington's disease might have trouble completing tasks when it becomes challenging to put thoughts together, or they might have difficulty adjusting to a sudden change in plans. Their symptoms can induce outbursts or make them seem uncooperative or apathetic. These are just some of the HD symptoms that impact relationships with family members and others. As Huntington's disease progresses, a person gradually loses their ability to speak, walk, and participate in daily life as they once did, and family members take on more of a caregiving role.

These ongoing changes take their toll on families. There are divorces and broken relationships in many HD families, and some people remove themselves from their families because of how difficult things become. This is scary for those who are at risk or gene positive because it is easy to worry about having a support network when it is needed most. For some families, though, these pressures bring family members closer together as they rely on each other to cope.

Relationships that are strained by the cognitive and behavioral symptoms of Huntington's disease can improve when HD symptoms change or become better managed. Ashley Clarke's relationship with her dad followed this pattern. When I first spoke with Ashley, her dad was living in a nursing home in Northern Ireland. As she shared her story, she described how their relationship changed over time.

Ashley was 15 years old and knew nothing about Huntington's disease when her dad was diagnosed, so she was shocked by the news. Ashley hadn't seen her dad in about nine months because his early HD symptoms had negatively affected their relationship. At the time, her family had little access to information about the disease. They were scared and unsure of how to handle the diagnosis or what to do next, but they did their best. Her parents were already divorced but remained good friends.

As Ashley described what her dad was like before he became symptomatic, she paused. "That's probably one of the hardest things," she said. "I can talk about my experience with HD until I am blue in the face. I love talking about it because it has become such a big part of my life and had such an impact. But the one thing that probably upsets me the most is I am getting to the point where I've nearly had a sick daddy longer than I had a healthy daddy." After Ashley learned her dad had Huntington's disease, she made a point of spending more time with him and making memories that would need to last a lifetime.

Ashley wishes she had had the opportunity to truly know her dad before he became symptomatic. When family and friends share stories about him, she thinks, "I never got to experience that daddy." Her dad loved water sports and had many trophies from water skiing events. "He was always up to devilment," she said. "If there was badness to get into, my daddy was in it. He was a great daddy. He was so much fun, and he was such a pillar of the community. Everybody knew him; everybody loved him; nobody had a bad word to say about him. He was one of the most hardworking men you've ever met."

After her dad's diagnosis, Ashley struggled in school even though she had always been a good student. She continued to work hard, though, and eventually moved an hour away from her hometown to attend college. Her dad started needing more care at this time. So, at the age of 17, Ashley attended college, held a job, and drove back and forth multiple times a week to make sure her dad had what he needed.

Ashley and her brother eventually worked out a system where her brother managed their dad's financial tasks and fixed anything that broke. Ashley managed their dad's medications, took him to appointments, and worked with the social workers. Managing her dad's care while attending school was stressful and required her to be ultra-organized with every day planned out. There was no wiggle room to accommodate any unexpected issues – something that is near impossible when caring for someone with Huntington's disease.

Coping with her dad's HD symptoms was challenging. Over time, Ashley learned to choose her battles and find creative solutions. She knew that if she tried to stop her dad from buying things he didn't need at the local shop, it could easily provoke an outburst, so she donated extra food to the local food bank. There were times she feared he might hit her, and she was injured more than once when trying to catch him as he fell. Each time, though, he had no recollection of what had happened by the next day. It was particularly important to Ashley that her dad looked presentable when they went out in public. It's common for those with symptomatic Huntington's disease to shower infrequently or appear disheveled. Ashley didn't want others to think her dad wasn't well cared for, so she helped him toilet, shower, and dress.

Ashley was often required to step out of her comfort zone to advocate for her dad, whether that meant negotiating with the local shop or battling with the social worker during routine visits. One social worker suggested Ashley and her brother weren't allowing their dad to make his own decision about a potential move to a nursing home. Ashley's dad struggled with remembering how to perform simple activities of daily living, so making a major life decision was more than he could process. "She ripped me apart and questioned everything I had done looking after him from when I was 17," Ashley said. "She got into my head. I started to believe what she was saying." Ashley's brother was worried about her, so she took a step back from caregiving. Her brother stepped in to fill the gap and wouldn't allow her to visit their dad for a while. Ashley needed a break.

Ashley's interactions with this particular social worker plus her dad's experience at an annual Orange Order parade – where paradegoers accused him of being drunk and called him a disgrace – prompted her to do something. "I knew nothing, and HDYO didn't exist," Ashley said. "There was nobody blogging about it; there was nobody writing about it. When you went to the internet, it was one horror story after another. If I can prevent that from happening to the younger generation coming behind me, that's all that's important to me." She started her own blog, called the *I'm Not Drunk Lifestyle Blog*, and openly shared about caring for her dad and her own testing journey.

When Ashley's dad moved to a nursing home, Ashley was able to focus more on her own life – something she hadn't done since her dad's diagnosis years earlier. When she visited her dad, they sat and talked and enjoyed their time together. This was a change from when he lived at home, and his daily care needs took precedence over spending quality time together. Ashley now has less to blog about related to her dad's daily care, so she shares lifestyle tips. She also shares tips from others who are caring for loved ones with Huntington's disease, such as how to increase calorie intake, using suspenders instead of a belt, or replacing shoes with foam clogs to make clean-up easier. She also helps others share their stories and does what she can to help people find the support they need.

One of Ashley's missions is to reduce the stigma around Huntington's disease, something she thinks is happening in the younger generation. "There's still a stigma about HD," she said, "but I think what I see in my generation, and the younger generation, is it's becoming more like: let's be kind about it, let's make people more aware, let's not hide our loved ones, let's not hide ourselves. I'm not a scientist – I can't go to a lab and create a cure – but I have a voice." Ashley sees a need to reduce stigma within the HD community as well. "I think we also need to change our perspectives and our opinions, and we need to talk about it more."

Ashley was obsessed with genetic testing after her dad's diagnosis. After all, she said, "My genes may be out to get me one day." She wanted to be prepared for her future, so it was hard to wait until she was 18 to get tested. She didn't know much about the testing process, so she was surprised that it would take months to get through all the genetic counseling appointments. She also didn't expect to encounter professionals' hesitancy to allow young adults to get tested. The social worker and genetic counselor questioned whether she should get tested while she was still in school. They also implied she was trying to get away from the responsibility of caring for her dad by going to a school an hour away from home, when in fact, she had chosen a school that allowed her to achieve her educational goals. What they didn't see was how hard she worked to make sure her dad received the care he needed, something that required her to regularly make the hourlong drive home to care for him.

As it neared time to draw blood for her genetic test, Ashley didn't feel like she had the professional support she needed from the social worker and counselor. She was also leaving soon to teach water sports in America for the summer. It seemed like a poor time to learn her gene status, so she waited. Her family and her local Northern Ireland HD charity helped her get through this difficult time. More than 10 years later, she still doesn't know her gene status. "Looking back," Ashley said, "I don't want to admit it, but I probably wasn't ready."

Ashley no longer feels the need to know. "Sometimes, I wish I got the result, just to have it over and done with and know my fate, and then other times, I don't really care," she said. "If I have it, I have it. If I don't, I don't. It's literally in my DNA, so I can't change it. I can't pop a pill and make it go away – not yet anyway! Knowing isn't going to help me. I'm young, I'm fit, I'm healthy. I mean, I don't want to get sick. I have an awesome life. I want to be snowboarding for another 50 years. I love my friends, I love my family, I love my life right now."

For Ashley, one of the hardest parts of Huntington's disease is that her dad became symptomatic when she was a teenager. She didn't get to hear her dad tell her, "Well done," for graduating university, learning a new trick on the wakeboard, or learning to fix her car. "I got it from my mum, my brother, my friends – but I never got it from him," Ashley said. "He's the one that I wanted it from the most. It's taken a lot to realize that I'm never going to get that. But I think if he was fit to speak now, he would say it."

Ashley has few pictures of her dad before he developed Huntington's disease. "I regret not taking more photos in the early days," she said. "In all the photos I have of me and daddy together – and I have a lot – he looks really sick. You would know he's in the late stages. He loves a wee photo, and he'll reach for my phone. I think he remembers me taking selfies with him, and he still wants that because why else is he reaching for my phone? Dad didn't know how to text; he didn't know what social media was, so he's not trying to check Facebook, you know."

Ashley's dad was unable to attend her university graduation, so Ashley and her family visited him immediately after the ceremony. She was still in her cap and gown. "We rushed down the road to daddy's nursing home," she said. "The staff had daddy in a suit, sitting at the door, waiting for me with a 'Congratulations!' balloon attached to his wheelchair. We had a cake. Mum got a present from her and daddy, and we had a graduation party." It was a first at the nursing home.

When her dad could no longer communicate, Ashley liked to imagine that in his mind, "He's at a drive-in movie theater, and he's sitting on a deck chair and watching all these wonderful memories – skiing and holidays and friends, and when my brother and I were born. And he's going, 'I had a pretty good life.' When we remember him and talk about him, we talk about all these fun, amazing memories – the stupid things he used to get up to." Whether or not she carries the expanded gene for Huntington's disease, Ashley hopes she can do the same someday. She hopes to live the kind of life where people will say, "'Geez, didn't Ashley do it all? Didn't she have a great life? Didn't she make some great memories?' I don't want people to say, 'Wasn't she a hard worker? Or didn't she have a nice house?' When you have that genetic fate hanging over you, I think it gives you a different outlook on life."

Ashley's dad passed away before she and I talked again one year later. "When Huntington's patients get to the stage that my dad was at, you're kind of waiting for it," she said. "You take every day as a blessing. Every time you say goodbye, you give a hug and a kiss because you don't know if that's going to be your last." Ashley and her brother were by their dad's side when he died. "I was there holding his hand," she said. "He wasn't alone; he wasn't scared. He knew he was loved because I told him every minute for the 10 days we were with him." Ashley feels blessed to have had the time she did with her dad.

Ashley's life has changed considerably since then. "The only way I can help people understand is to imagine having a two-year-old kid, and you have to do everything for that kid," she explained. "They are the light and life of your soul, and everything you do is to make them proud and make sure they have everything they need – food, clothes, your love, your time. Then, all of a sudden, they aren't there. So, what do I do now? I'm trying to find where I belong because I'm no longer a carer."

Ashley continues to advocate for the HD community, including serving as a member of HD-CAB and the HDYO board. She's also taking up hobbies, like learning to play the bagpipes and landing the lead role in a local play. After Ashley's dad died, someone told her that her dad had left her a legacy to continue raising awareness of Huntington's disease. "That's so true," Ashley said. "I have this opportunity – this platform – to help people." Over time, Ashley's relationship with her dad changed from one that was strained by her dad's HD symptoms and the stresses of providing care to a relationship that inspires her to carry his legacy forward.

Now that I've seen my brother's HD progression, I understand why things were so difficult for my dad, and why I found him hard to relate to. Having missed a chance to understand and know my dad before he died, I know how important it is to maintain a relationship with my brother, even though that's not easy. When I visit my brother, it's hard to have a conversation with him. There's no natural give-and-take, something that reminds me of conversations I had with my dad. It's especially hard when I visit by myself and there aren't other family members to help fill in the gaps.

My brother can provide simple answers to questions, but he is unable to ask his own questions in return or initiate a new thread to a conversation. Talking to him can feel lopsided, but we manage. He likes it when I talk about the past. If I remind him about something from our childhood or his early adult years, he remembers and will say something like "Oh yeah!" Every now and then, we find other ways to communicate, like when he looked at me expectantly in the middle of dinner and burped loudly – twice – with a big smile on his face. I'm sure it was for my benefit. It was his way of playfully reaching out and saying hello.

On a recent visit to see my brother and his family, I delivered a box stuffed with items my mom saved over the years. When I dropped it off, I didn't realize what a treasure trove it contained. As my brother and his family explored the box's contents, my brother's family learned new things about him and his life experiences. There were newspaper clippings about the activities he was involved in during high school, letters he wrote home about meeting my sister-in-law along with later letters about wanting to marry her, and postcards from his travels around the world.

The contents allow my brother to share things about his life now that he can no longer share them himself. The box is full of memories and conversation starters that help his family learn about a younger version of my brother. Instead of being a sad reminder of what has been lost, though, the box provides a fun way for my brother and his family to connect with each other. Sharing these experiences together allows my brother to contribute to the conversation in his own way.

TALKING ABOUT HUNTINGTON'S DISEASE

Once I learned I was at risk for Huntington's disease, I had to go through a process of *becoming* at risk. I had to sort through and internalize a lot of complex emotions before I could even consider sharing my experience with others. This took time. For several years, I was uncomfortable talking about Huntington's disease, even with family members. I rarely brought it up in conversation with friends because I knew talking about it would require a lot of explanation, something I wasn't good at in the early days when I was still learning about the disease. Talking about common symptoms and care became easier over time, but describing my feelings and fears did not. I didn't know how to bridge the gap to help people understand the nuances of this family disease, so I often felt alone as I came to terms with my at-risk status. I felt like I had a secret life with vastly different worries than those of the people around me.

At the time of my brother's diagnosis, I already had a long history of not talking about my family. My HD story unknowingly began when I met my grandpa in a psychiatric hospital, and it continued when I witnessed my dad's mental health struggles. Talking about mental health at that time was still taboo, so I hesitated to tell others what was happening at home. I didn't want people to judge me or my family. Even now, my natural tendency is to direct conversation away from myself. I don't know if this is an inherent part of my personality or a defense mechanism I adopted to avoid telling people about my family. I suspect it's a little of both. Regardless, I was accustomed to not sharing big parts of my life long before I knew about Huntington's disease. There are people I've known for years – decades even – who knew nothing about my experiences with my dad and grandpa.

Telling people about my brother's diagnosis and my newly revealed at-risk status forced me to share my thoughts, feelings, and experiences. I was selective in who I told and what I shared because I worried people might think about me differently if they knew I was at risk for this disease. I didn't want others to analyze me or my mannerisms to determine if I was showing symptoms. I didn't want anyone to have a reason to doubt me or my abilities. I was surrounded by supportive friends and family who did not judge me, but these were some of my worries, nonetheless. Once I tested negative, I became a little more comfortable talking about Huntington's disease. When I started my conversations with the HD community, my comfort grew with each interaction – something for which I am grateful. Practice has helped immensely.

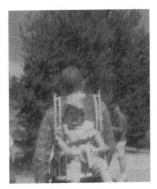

My dad loved to explore the outdoors and made sure we experienced nature from an early age.

Stigma stifles openness

Stigma refers to negative feelings, false beliefs, or prejudices people have about another person's characteristics, circumstances, or health symptoms. The stigma that surrounds Huntington's disease has created what some call a culture of silence, and Huntington's disease is a family secret for many. Stigma can affect a person's willingness to disclose their HD gene status or seek support, and it can lead to caregiver and patient isolation. Stigma can also have a negative impact on the quality of care our loved ones receive. Advocacy and education efforts in recent years have increased people's comfort with talking about illness, mental illness, and disability, but stigma still exists.

Deciding whether to reveal or withhold your HD gene status is a complicated personal decision with real-world implications. Potential consequences of sharing include being shunned by others, facing discrimination in the workplace, or losing access to some kinds of insurance in certain countries. In the United States, the Affordable Care Act ensures that health insurance cannot be denied due to pre-existing conditions, but it is still difficult, if not impossible, to get life insurance and long-term care insurance if you are at risk or gene positive. The Genetic Information Nondiscrimination Act is another US policy that prevents employers from requiring employees to disclose their gene status for any genetic disease. While employees cannot be terminated for disclosing their gene status, they can be let go if they have symptoms that prevent them from performing their job duties.

Unfortunately, workplace discrimination still exists despite these protections. Not long before her mom passed away, one *Livable Lives* storyteller was asked by her employer to explain why her personal struggles were impacting her work performance. Her employer knew she was caring for her mom who was in poor health but didn't know her mom had Huntington's disease. When this storyteller explained her mom's condition, she disclosed that she had tested positive herself but didn't expect to become symptomatic for decades. Her employer let her go because she was still in the probationary period for her job. Her employer didn't want to fully train someone who would not have a "long-term commitment with their company." She was furious. When she reached out to her local HD organization, she learned that she was under no obligation to reveal her gene status to an employer, nor did she have to tell them she will be disabled one day.

Many people in the HD community share their stories despite any risks that doing so might carry. This is especially true for Megha Bhaduri, a gene-positive young woman who is making a documentary film about her family's HD experience. Megha wants to raise awareness of Huntington's disease in her home country of India where the disease is highly stigmatized. When we spoke, Megha had known for five years that she is gene positive. She is the only person in her family who has confirmed her gene status through genetic testing, but her dad and grandfather both had the disease.

Megha knew nothing about Huntington's disease growing up. The first time she heard of it was when she was in college and returned home for a visit. She was using her dad's laptop and saw a letter to his boss about using his accumulated medical leave to retire early. The letter mentioned Huntington's disease, so she looked it up. Her dad's symptoms suddenly made sense, and Megha had to come to terms with the gravity of her dad's illness and her own at-risk status.

When Megha told a childhood friend about her dad's illness, her friend was surprised Megha didn't realize other people knew her dad was sick. Megha herself didn't realize how sick he was until she spent time away from him. "I don't think I was dealing with it very well mentally," she said. "Every time I went home, he was sicker. When I was living with him, I didn't see those changes. When I went away for three months, six months – it was daunting to see how sick he was getting. The only people I could speak to at that point were my friends." Megha and her friends learned about Huntington's disease together. "It was always open communication with them first, before I even tried communicating with my family," she said.

The family nature of Huntington's disease stands out to Megha. "Something that people need to understand about Huntington's is how complicated the whole family structure of it is. I grew up seeing a very sick parent and a sick family around me, and I could never speak about it," she said. "My father grew up seeing the same things with his dad, and when I have symptoms, my children will grow up seeing the same things. Any amount of empathy would go a long way."

Megha thinks parents have an obligation not only to help their children understand the disease, but also to become their ally and create a family support system. "If they never told me what Huntington's was, and I happened to find out in school from somebody, and maybe the first few words thrown around were that the person looks drunk or the person is crazy… If that's how I'm perceiving my father," she said, "then I'm not a support system for him. Everybody needs to be a support system to the families, children included. I think the more knowledge you have about it, the easier you can navigate it."

Before Megha's dad got sick, he was very sociable. "He could crack people up and make a lot of jokes," she said. "Most people knew him as a walking, talking encyclopedia, so he was a fun person to be around. I think he instilled this sense of wanting to learn in both me and my brother, making sure that we were quizzing on a regular basis, making sure we were going through the atlas or the encyclopedias. I remember that aspect of him well. After he fell sick, a lot of that went." Megha still loves to learn, and she continues to enjoy maps, studying history, and traveling.

Megha was 12 or 13 years old when her dad started exhibiting what she now knows were early HD symptoms. "It started with a lot of emotional upheavals," she said. "It was evident that he was depressed, and he was anxious. He had psychosis and OCD, but I couldn't understand any of those things at that point. He felt like a distant father in my teenage years. There was a lot of tension in the house because he would react to things in, I would say, violent ways. I don't think I had a safe environment growing up." Megha used to blame her dad for how difficult home life became, and she stopped talking to him for a long time. Now, though, she knows that her dad's HD symptoms were not his fault. Megha's dad died when she was 22.

Megha's brother had a different experience. Her brother is older, so he got to spend more time with their dad before he developed symptoms, and he remembers their grandfather who passed away before Megha was born. Their parents didn't talk to Megha about what was happening to their dad, but they did talk to her brother. They thought he was more emotionally stable than Megha. For all these reasons, Megha thinks her brother had a deeper relationship with their father.

Being at risk was hard for Megha. She's always been a planner and prefers to know her next five steps in life, so she decided to get tested for Huntington's disease. "I felt the emotional upheaval of it and the psychological symptoms of it," she said. "I felt like I was likely to have Huntington's. I was also of the mind that I would not be able to rest if I didn't know if I had it or not." Megha's mother also thought it was likely Megha was gene positive and discouraged her from getting tested.

Megha was familiar with genetic testing protocols in the United States and the United Kingdom, so she expected to undergo a similar months-long period of genetic counseling when she started her own testing journey. When her genetic counselor mentioned going to the lab during her first appointment, Megha thought they were just going to take a look. "I was being really naïve," she said. "I ended up going to the lab and they took my blood. I could not understand what was happening. They said they'd get back to me in three days. I had no time to prepare for what was coming. I consider myself lucky that I had spent a couple of years telling myself that it could be something I had. If I had just gone into it without any understanding, and if I didn't have the support system that I had, I don't think I would have handled the result very well."

Learning that she is gene positive didn't take away many of the questions Megha had hoped would be answered by knowing her gene status. "While it's nice to know that something is going to happen," she said, "I don't know exactly what's going to happen, at what time, and what the progression is going to be. It still leaves me in the dark, which is not what I wanted." She sometimes questions whether getting tested was the right or wrong decision. "I could have easily lived without knowing that I have Huntington's, but it's also helped in a way. I don't want to hold myself back from doing things that somebody else might think they'd do in 10 years, because I don't know what I'll be like in 10 years. It's allowed me to make decisions and value the space I'm in a little more. But I still don't know if I made the right decision."

Several of Megha's family members do not believe that Huntington's disease is part of their genetic heritage. As the only person in her family who knows her gene status, it is easy to feel isolated. "I feel lonely in the whole process because I don't feel like anyone in my family understands what it's like to have Huntington's," Megha said. "The only person who would have understood was my dad, and he's not around. No matter how much I try and explain myself to my mom or my grandma or my friends, and however hard they try, they'll never completely understand what's going on in my head. It would have been nice to have had a slightly more open relationship with my dad, so I felt more prepared for what's to come."

Thinking about how her disease will progress is overwhelming. "I know I have the psychological symptoms," Megha said. "If somebody gave me the option of choosing only the physical or only the psychological symptoms of Huntington's, I think I would always pick the physical ones. I know I might not be walking, and I might be in a wheelchair – and that would frustrate the living daylights out of me – but I still would have a working, functioning brain. My brain feels foggy. I'm just 28, so I don't even know what it will be like in the future. It's very daunting. I know that it's just going to keep getting worse."

Time passes much too quickly for Megha, and she often feels sad on her birthday or when a new year begins. Five years ago, she thought she had a lot of time before symptoms would appear, but those five years have flown by. "If my next 10 years go by at the speed of the last five years, will I be able to achieve enough in my life?" she asked. "I know I tested exactly for this reason, where I could tell myself, 'Okay, you only have 10 years. Somebody else might have 30 years, but you have 10 years, so scrunch everything together.' But I can't do everything in a short period of time, and I hate having been dealt the bad hand in this situation."

After living in the United States for several years as a student, Megha considered staying. She knows she doesn't want to be in India when she develops more symptoms. The Indian healthcare system is not set up to serve HD patients well, and there is a significant lack of knowledge even within the medical community. When she attended an HD event in India, for example, she was surprised to hear doctors' answers to questions from the audience. "There was no understanding of it being genetic; there was no understanding of it being degenerative," she said. Even so, Megha is hopeful that India's medical community will continue to expand its understanding of Huntington's disease and develop more services and care facilities for the HD community.

Megha finds hope in a future that might provide better options for medications and healthcare, but she has more hope for the next generation than her own. For herself, she finds hope in doing what she can to live an independent life as long as possible, hopefully into her 30s and 40s. Megha doesn't talk to her mom about Huntington's disease on purpose. "She had to deal with my dad for so many years, and it was hard enough for her," Megha said. "The assumption is that she is going to be my primary caregiver in the next couple of years. I would like to give her a couple of years of respite." To take her mind off things and keep from spiraling downward, Megha takes long walks in nature and listens to music. She also finds a lot of support from HDYO and online HD groups. She has volunteered for the Huntington's Society of India, and she's involved in HDYO and HD-CAB. She also takes advantage of opportunities to speak publicly about the disease.

When Megha started her documentary, she originally planned to include other HD families. One of the biggest challenges Megha has faced while working on her film is that people in India do not talk about illness, especially mental illness. Talking openly about Huntington's disease can jeopardize access to healthcare or result in a loss of health insurance. HD families rarely tell people outside the family about the disease, and many don't even talk openly amongst themselves. They are more likely to say a loved one has depression.

While researching her film, Megha met two Indian families with very different HD experiences. She encountered the rare example of a 75-year-old woman who was surrounded by people who understood Huntington's disease. Her home was set up to accommodate her needs, including cushioning throughout the house to protect her if she fell. "The house was so emotionally stable, and nobody was getting frustrated. Everyone understood how to live with her," Megha said. "I believe she's one of the happiest patients I've ever seen."

Megha encountered a different story when she met with a mother and two sons, one of whom had Juvenile Huntington's disease. The father had died of Huntington's disease several years earlier, and no one in their small town understood the disease. "The community believed it was contagious, so they wouldn't come near the family," Megha said. "They wouldn't eat at their house; they wouldn't talk to them; they wouldn't touch them. I had no idea there was such a lack of knowledge." Due to the stigma attached to Huntington's disease in India, families that initially agreed to be part of her documentary decided not to participate. The film now features Megha's family alone.

When Megha releases her film, she wants it to be seen throughout India. Along with the film, she plans to distribute children's books and educational materials translated into the languages of each region. After growing up with no knowledge of the disease, she hopes her film and educational materials will help young people understand Huntington's disease and cope better with belonging to an HD family. Sharing her family's story will make a difference and add to the momentum that already exists to further reduce the stigma surrounding Huntington's disease.

Talking with children

I have only a vague recollection of what I said when I told my boys that my brother had Huntington's disease and the three of us were at risk. I told them not long after my brother's diagnosis, when I was still in shock and processing this significant change in our lives. I was just starting to learn about the disease, so I hadn't yet mastered the major talking points. If my family had known about Huntington's disease before my dad died, I likely would have thought about how to have this conversation for years before it happened. I had yet to come across articles about what to consider when talking to kids about Huntington's disease, so I simply followed my intuition. My boys were 13 and 16 years old at the time, so I felt they were old enough to learn about the disease's genetic component.

If I had taken more time to think about how to tell my kids about Huntington's disease, I might have chosen different words. I think I would have told them a little at a time over several conversations instead of everything all at once. Even if I had known more before this conversation, I still might have second-guessed my approach simply because what I had to tell them changed everything. In a way, this conversation marked an end to their innocence – an end to assuming their future held only possibility. This conversation introduced them to my mortality and theirs. In the years between this conversation and receiving my negative genetic test result, I asked my boys many times if they had questions or wanted to talk through their concerns. They always assured me they were doing okay. My absence of symptoms kept their worries at bay, but not mine, and I continued to be concerned about how they were coping.

Conversations with children build the foundation for how they perceive the disease and its effects on their family and themselves, as well as how they will one day approach their own gene status. Deciding when and how to tell children about Huntington's disease, and especially its genetic component, is a complicated decision, and there is no perfect time. HD organizations provide many resources to help with these conversations, including guidance for parents and age-appropriate explanations for children. A good rule of thumb is to provide an environment where children feel comfortable sharing their thoughts and letting their questions guide the conversation. It is important that children learn about Huntington's disease from family members or trusted sources, instead of learning about it from people who don't understand the disease or from sources that may not provide the age-appropriate explanation they need.

Children are often more aware of what is happening in their family than parents realize, and children may recognize early on that there's something unusual about an HD family member. To make sense of the situation, a child may create their own explanation, or they may worry excessively or feel responsible for causing the changes they see. Children who are introduced to Huntington's disease early may be less likely to misinterpret a family member's HD symptoms, especially their behavioral symptoms. It may be easier for them to maintain a positive relationship with an HD family member instead of becoming angry with or afraid of them. Many parents decide to tell young children that a family member has Huntington's disease but wait until children are older to tell them about the genetic component.

It is important for children to know that others share or understand their experiences. Two *Livable Lives* storytellers specifically mentioned an HDYO YouTube video called, *Huntington's Disease – The Impact on Young People*, in which young people describe what it's like to grow up in an HD family. For both, this video often felt like their only connection to someone who understood, and they watched it over and over. Other storytellers mentioned that their parents educated family, friends, and neighbors about Huntington's disease to create a support network around them. Knowing that others understood what their family was going through made it easier to talk about Huntington's disease and cope with belonging to an HD family.

Several *Livable Lives* storytellers grew up in families that talk openly about Huntington's disease, so they were aware of it from a young age. Others clearly remember learning about the disease for the first time. Experiences varied widely – some good, and some bad. Bailey Pratt is an at-risk young woman from New York whose mom created a safe and supportive environment for her to learn about and talk about Huntington's disease. Their conversations have helped Bailey feel like she has a reliable safety net even though her future is uncertain.

Bailey was very young when she learned her dad had Huntington's disease. She doesn't remember feeling shocked by the news. "My mom did a great job explaining to us what was going on," Bailey said. "I was seven or eight, and she told us, 'Your dad is sick. He has things going on in his brain – things we can't control. He can go to doctors, and they can help him out. But from our point of view, we love him the same – we treat him the same – no matter what's going on in his head that he can't control.' The way she explained it didn't scare me." Several years later, Bailey's mom felt it was time to tell Bailey and her older sister they were at risk, but she didn't know how. A social worker came to the house to start this difficult conversation, and then Bailey's mom took it from there.

Bailey's mom repeatedly reassures her daughters that she will always be there for them. "She tells me, 'I want you to live life to your full potential. Do what makes you happy and do it every day. I don't want you to regret anything. Everything's going to be just fine whether you carry this gene or not.' That takes weight off my shoulders," Bailey said. "Being at risk, I worry about who's going to take care of me. I don't want to burden anybody because I know how difficult that is. When I look at my mom, I don't think that she would ever feel any type of burden or guilt about having to do that. She's definitely made it as easy as it can be by carrying that weight of not knowing what's going to happen in the future."

Bailey has few memories of her dad before he developed Huntington's disease. He was a Marine and a police officer. He used to ride motorcycles, ski, snowboard, mountain bike – anything to be active. Bailey thinks her mom and older sister shielded her from knowing about some of her dad's early HD symptoms, like excessive drinking and difficulty managing finances. There are other things she thinks she has chosen to forget. Still, she has plenty of good memories of her dad. Bailey's close friends always knew about her dad's disease, and she didn't hesitate to invite them over. "All of my close friends were comfortable with it. I was comfortable with it; he was comfortable with it. We never hid him, ever," she said. "He was always involved in everything we had going on. I think it was as normal as it could have been."

Bailey's parents were divorced, so there were times when Bailey helped her grandma care for her dad. "I would feed my dad from time to time," Bailey said, "but it made me anxious because he choked a lot. At the same time, it broke my heart. I was only 15 or 16 and feeding my dad." Her anxiety turned to fear after she witnessed one extreme choking episode. "Thank God, his nurse was there. His eyes were literally coming out of his face, and his lips were blue. I didn't know what to do. Ever since then, I was like, I'm not feeding him. 'I love you dad, but I'm not doing that.'"

As soon as Bailey and her older sister were old enough, Bailey's mom connected them with HDYO. The sisters attended an HDYO camp in California several years ago. "Having that group of people changed my whole life," Bailey said. "Knowing other people feel this way helped a lot growing up." Bailey found comfort in talking to others who had similar experiences, and she continues to find support through the relationships she built there. While Bailey and her sister weren't in the same group at camp, this shared experience made it easier for the two sisters to talk about Huntington's disease. "I think that brought us very close together. We're close as it is, but we sat down and talked about things." They are now better equipped to talk about how belonging to an HD family affects them.

Still, there are days when talking about Huntington's disease is the last thing Bailey wants to do. "I'm tired of this being in my life," she said. "I don't know if it's ever going to go away. Everyone in my life who has had Huntington's has passed away, but I still have two sisters and myself. My younger sister wants to talk about it all the time. But some days, I don't want to."

Bailey has had mixed experiences when talking about Huntington's disease with people outside the HD community. When she used to tell people her dad was sick, she was often met with replies of, "Just stay positive," or "Have hope – he'll get better." These responses made her angry. She typically responded with, "No... he won't... but thank you." She knows most people don't know what Huntington's disease is, but she wishes they had at least a little understanding.

Bailey has seen several therapists in recent years, but she has yet to find one who understands the nuances of Huntington's disease. They focused on her dad and his disease when she needed help coping with her own at-risk status. One therapist said things like, "I was like that when I was your age," or "That happens to everybody." Bailey found this frustrating – the therapist didn't get it. Bailey's experience highlights the importance of finding the right therapist – a therapist who is a good fit and who knows, or at least tries, to understand what it means to belong to an HD family.

One of Bailey's friends isn't from an HD family, but she is empathetic in a way that makes Bailey feel understood. When Bailey told this friend her dad was sick, but it was hard to explain, the friend asked for an explanation – she wanted to know. This friend also notices when Bailey seems down and asks how she's feeling. "When we talk about college," Bailey said, "she's open with talking about how maybe a certain path could be better for my future, or things like that. I'm comfortable around her. I think seeing things from someone else's perspective helps, even though they might not understand 100 percent."

For Bailey, the hardest part of Huntington's disease is, "Watching somebody you love start to disappear... They're there, but they're not. It was difficult growing up and not being 100 percent sure who my dad was before he got sick. I have a lot of jealousy of my mom and my aunt because they got to see him as the person he was meant to be, and I never got to see that." Bailey's dad passed away in 2020 moments after she landed at the airport but before she was able to get to him. She's angry that he died before she got to tell him goodbye in person. "I was literally on my way," she said. "At the same time, I can stop worrying about him. I miss him every single day. I wish he had had a different life, but I know we did all we could to make it as normal as possible. I find comfort in knowing that he was a very positive role model in my life despite having Huntington's. He was never resentful. I look up to him, for sure."

Being at risk shapes how Bailey thinks about her future. "I definitely think being at risk has changed a lot of views in my life," she said, "but in a positive way." When making important life decisions, she thinks about what would be best for her if she were to have Huntington's disease, rather than feeling like her life will be over if she has it. "There are definitely times where all I can think is negative thoughts, but I think that's how it is with anybody with Huntington's disease." Bailey doesn't plan to get tested. "I don't think I want to put myself in that position," she said. "I struggle with anxiety as it is. I've gotten comfortable with the idea of not knowing. Who knows what's going to happen in your life despite being at risk for something? I would rather live every day like any other person who doesn't know what's going to happen in their future."

When a friend tested positive for Huntington's disease, it reinforced Bailey's decision to remain at risk. "I saw her world crash. It was emotional for me to see somebody go through that, knowing that my father went through that, and my grandfather went through that," Bailey said. "I don't want to put myself through that, because I don't know if I could handle it. As much as it burdens me – literally every day of my life – I feel more comfortable not knowing. I have people who are going to be there for me and love me regardless." Bailey has learned a lot from belonging to an HD family. "As difficult as Huntington's disease is, it has opened my world in so many ways," she said. "Being closer as a family, for one. I just wish our family wasn't glued together by Huntington's disease."

Difficult conversations

Talking about Huntington's disease can be very difficult. As members of a rare disease community, we have to decide over and over whether to reveal we belong to an HD family, and we have to decide when, who, and how much to tell. Some of our experiences are too painful to put into words, so there is often much more to our stories than what we share publicly. Many of us only share in situations where we feel safe, like after knowing someone for a considerable amount of time. When we do share, we might find ourselves reassuring the people we're talking to that we're okay – we can manage, we're strong – when in fact, that may not always be true.

Even with society's growing openness and willingness to discuss disease and mental health, we often gloss over many details of our HD stories. We might focus on the bigger events, but sometimes day-to-day life is just as difficult. Take my brother for instance. Over several years, he changed from an easygoing and fun-loving guy to a person with behavioral and cognitive symptoms that led to an involuntary stay in a psychiatric ward. A lot happened along the way. As my husband said, "It culminated in this big event, but the train was wrecking for a long time."

Sometimes, when we share our stories, others tell us to have hope or assure us everything will be okay. "A cure will be found in time," they might say, or "Anyone can get hit by a bus on any given day. We all live with risk." These responses feel dismissive and reflect a lack of understanding about Huntington's disease, its effects on individuals and families, and the fear the disease can instill. Take the getting-hit-by-a-bus example. It's true that everyone lives with risk. Knowing that we're all going to die someday is no surprise, but almost no one seriously contemplates getting hit by a bus when they walk out their front door each morning. In the HD community, however, a future with Huntington's disease is not hypothetical. It's very real. The odds of getting hit by a bus are nearly nonexistent compared to the 50-50 chance of having Huntington's disease if you're at risk or the certainty of having it if you're gene positive. The chances of getting hit by a bus and having Huntington's disease cannot be compared.

Researchers have found that many people in HD families do not share much about their experiences, in part because there's a fear of letting people in, and in part because there's a fear that others will be judgmental or won't understand. Keeping this information close can prevent relationships from deepening, and many people experience loneliness and isolation when those around them know little about the disease. Mallory is an at-risk young woman from Colorado who has struggled with whether and when to share her HD experiences, something that has affected her relationships with friends.

Mallory was in high school when her dad was diagnosed with Huntington's disease, a disease her family knew nothing about. Learning she was at risk changed everything at a time when she had been eagerly thinking about college, a career, and her adult identity. Mallory's initial response was to avoid the subject altogether. She remembers telling family members to stop talking to her about Huntington's disease. They couldn't do anything about it, and she needed to just live her life. When Mallory went to college, she compartmentalized her life and tried not to think about Huntington's disease, her own at-risk status, and what was happening back home. "I definitely lived at college as if this wasn't happening," she said. She thinks it took at least three years to fully process and incorporate Huntington's disease into her life.

After her dad's diagnosis, family and friends would ask Mallory how her dad was doing, and then they would ask how her mom was doing. It made her angry that they never went one step further and asked how she was doing. She sometimes thinks her at-risk status represents a lot of the sadness associated with Huntington's disease: she's losing a parent to the disease, and she's facing the possibility of having the disease herself someday. That's a lot for other people to understand.

Deciding whether and how much to tell her friends about Huntington's disease has not been easy. During high school and college, she told a few close friends about her dad's diagnosis, but only after they reached best-friend status. Even with her best friends, sharing her story was overwhelming. Mallory eventually learned there are layers of sharing. The first layer is telling people her dad is sick and sharing information about the symptoms of the disease. She often stops there because she already feels vulnerable.

The next layer is revealing that the disease is genetic, something she doesn't feel comfortable sharing. Talking about being at risk makes her emotionally distraught and reinforces how alone she feels. "One of the hardest things about Huntington's disease has been that disconnect where I feel like I'm going through something so difficult that I can't even process it and share it with other people," she said. "When I do share with other people, it almost makes that disconnect bigger."

When Mallory first opened up to friends, many didn't know how to react, so they didn't say anything at all. She ended up feeling worse after sharing. Other friends responded immediately with questions about her future. Will she get tested? Will she get married someday? Is she going to have kids? How does being at risk affect her career goals? While these may seem like natural questions to ask, they are extremely personal and jarring to Mallory. "Thinking about my future is just a little more complicated," she said. She feels torn between telling her friends what they expect to hear (that she has big plans for her future despite the obstacles) or an honest answer (that every decision is affected by her gene status). Being asked these questions makes Mallory uncomfortable, even though she thinks about these things all the time.

It took Mallory a while to realize why telling friends about Huntington's disease made her feel sadder. "I felt like I was keeping this big secret," she said, "so I expected that telling them would alleviate my suffering. When I finally did tell them, there was still so much pain – the pain of having a sick dad and being at risk. Telling my friends about HD didn't solve those problems. At the end of the day, telling friends doesn't get rid of HD, but sharing helps me process and live authentically without compartmentalizing so much."

Since finishing college and moving back to her hometown, Mallory has been seeing her family on a regular basis. "Huntington's disease is much more integrated into my life now, so I want to be more open with people early on," she said. "I'm realizing that I get to choose what I do and don't share about HD." She finds this new mindset empowering, which is a good change from the days when thoughts about Huntington's disease ruled her life.

Mallory is much more comfortable talking about Huntington's disease now. "I feel like I've grown, and things have changed in the past year," she said. "Many of my friends have learned how to talk about HD, and I've learned how to share what I need to. I've had many conversations where I end up feeling so grateful for the people in my life who amaze me with how compassionate and caring they are. When I talk about the hard stuff with certain friends, I feel so safe and supported by them that I end up crying because I'm so overwhelmed."

Mallory recently told a new friend at work about her dad but stopped short of sharing her own at-risk status. When this new friend asked a series of questions that made Mallory feel like she might understand in a way others hadn't before, however, Mallory felt more comfortable opening up. This new friend asked questions about the bigger impacts of Huntington's disease, like Mallory's dad's day-to-day life, the progression of his disease, how Mallory and her family are coping, and whether Mallory is close to her dad. "One of her early questions was whether my dad is depressed," Mallory said. "I don't feel like anyone has ever asked me that before and considered my dad's mental health. I was struck by how kind and humanizing her question was. It showed me just how much she was listening and cared."

For Mallory, one of the saddest parts of Huntington's disease is the impact on her relationship with her dad, a relationship that became strained by her dad's HD symptoms when Mallory was a teenager. She likes to reminisce about camping trips they took together when she was small. Mallory shares her dad's love for camping, hiking, and traveling, so she wonders if she and her dad would still be going on adventures together if he could. "It's a confusing feeling, where I miss someone who is still here," she said. "I don't know the healthy, happy, vibrant version of my dad that other people tell me about. I don't know what aspects of my dad are *him*, and what aspects are *his disease*. I struggle with the thought that I know the HD version of my dad, but I don't know him. Does that mean if I have HD someday, I will lose myself?"

Mallory wishes she could have a conversation with her dad so she could ask questions to better understand him. She'd like to know what it's like to have Huntington's disease. Does his brain feel different? Does he feel like himself? She could ask these questions now, but he wouldn't be able to give any details in his answer. She wonders if asking him would be cruel, but she's curious to know what he's feeling so she can better understand what might lie ahead for herself.

Mallory thinks her family has become closer because of their HD journey, but in a different way than if Huntington's disease wasn't part of their lives. Mallory sometimes finds it difficult to manage her own response to Huntington's disease while trying to support her family. "I wish I had more emotional energy," she said. "I feel like we're all stretched so thin, and I don't know how to help everyone." Mallory realizes she needs to deal with the disease a little at a time. For now, she focuses on her dad and her family. "There's so much going on with my dad that is hard and stressful and sad, but it is also the part of HD that I know and understand. I know what's going to happen to him. I know it's going to be hard, but there are things that I can do to help him get better care, and support my mom, and help my family through this."

While belonging to an HD family has been tough, Mallory has learned that she has more control over her life than she used to think she did. "If I want to be a happy and positive person, and if I want to enjoy my life and have meaningful relationships and bring joy to others' lives, I can do that," she said. "I can also not do that. It's totally up to me. Other people want to see me be happy, but they can't do anything about that. That's all my responsibility and my privilege to do that for myself. If I'm angry that none of my friends are asking me how I'm doing, I can't control that. But if I have something I want to share with them, all I have to do is share. Realizing I have free choice, even though I don't have a choice about HD, has been empowering."

Mallory's relationship to Huntington's disease changed when she decided to get more involved in the HD community. She had a transformational experience when she attended an HD youth camp and connected with other young adults from HD families. She met an amazing group of people and felt like it was the first time she was grateful to have Huntington's disease in her life. On the first evening, she sat for several hours with a group of peers talking, sharing, and sobbing. "I can't even describe how cool that was," she said, "to have had such a painful and terrible thing happen in my family where my whole experience was dominated by feeling like no one understood – not even my close people. Meeting new people who put into words what I had been feeling and who understood exactly what I was saying – I'd never experienced anything like that. It was one of the coolest nights of my life. That type of community was the most wonderful, healing, helpful experience ever."

Sharing our HD stories is emotional. Starting the conversation is difficult because it is hard to know how much to reveal, and there is no predicting how others will respond. Even those who are comfortable sharing their HD story publicly may continue to keep their most painful experiences private, and that's okay. It's not necessary to be an open book. Sharing our stories can be as simple as having a personal conversation with the people around us to help them understand the challenges of belonging to an HD family.

While talking about Huntington's disease is not easy, I want to draw attention to a very important point that emerged in my conversations with the HD community: with the right people, at the right time, and in a supportive environment, talking about Huntington's disease can have amazing outcomes. It can help a child understand what they see happening around them, it can help someone who is at risk or gene positive feel like they have support as they face their future, and it can help members of the HD community feel like they are not alone. Ultimately, sharing our experiences can reduce stigma and increase compassion, understanding, and support for HD families, all of which can contribute to a more livable life for the HD community.

RESOURCES

FINDING SOMEONE TO TALK TO

If you are having a difficult time or need support, please seek help from a family member, a friend, a therapist, a faith leader, or emergency services. If you need help finding someone to talk to about Huntington's disease, reach out to an HD organization. Most HD organizations provide online and in-person support groups, and most have social workers or other staff who can help you directly or connect you to another source of support.

In addition, it can be helpful to see how others talk about the difficulties of living with Huntington's disease. The HDYO website includes a video series called, *Breaking Down Barriers*, in which participants talk about issues like gene status, genetic testing, caregiving, stigma, suicide, and much more.

TALKING WITH CHILDREN ABOUT HUNTINGTON'S DISEASE

The HDYO website has many resources for talking with children. In addition to a *Breaking Down Barriers* video on the subject, check out their YouTube video titled, *Huntington's Disease – The Impact on Young People*. The HDYO website also includes a section called, *HD Land*, that helps children under age 12 understand Huntington's disease.

In addition, HD Reach and the UC Davis Health System's HDSA Center of Excellence both have guides on their websites for talking with children about Huntington's disease.

OUTLOOK ON LIFE

Learning I was at risk for Huntington's disease changed how I defined myself and how I envisioned my future. I thought about what lay ahead much more than I ever had before. I had seen how the disease affected my brother, my dad, and my grandpa, and I had to reconcile myself to a future in which those around me might no longer be able to connect with the person I am today. It was rare to have a day when I didn't think about two conflicting versions of myself: one that would have Huntington's disease, and one that would not. Instead of feeling like I had an uncertain future, it felt more like my future was very defined. I just didn't know which version it was going to be. It took time, but I eventually adopted a new way of thinking about my life that included these two contrasting versions of my future self.

When I tested negative, and my future became known, I didn't return to being the person I was before I knew about Huntington's disease. That person is long gone. Once again, I had to redefine myself and my approach to life. Since then, my intense focus on the future has eased, but the gene-positive life I had to consider is not gone. I thought testing negative would free me from that life, but it lingers as a counterpoint to the life I get to live. There's a balancing act that takes place in my mind where I still compare these two versions. Knowing what my life might have been gives me a greater appreciation for the many good things in my life. Supporting my brother and his family is of utmost importance, and I want to devote myself to things that contribute to the greater good. I've gained an important perspective about what's important to me, and I am always aware that my life could have been different.

Many people in the HD community have this same dual view of the future, and many who have gone through the testing process also find that learning their HD gene status requires a shift in how they define themselves and their outlook on life. It's a perpetual identity crisis:

- If you're *at risk*, your identity has a hidden component – a part of yourself that is very real and present but unknown;
- If you're *gene positive but presymptomatic*, your identity includes a future self that will be very different from who you are today;
- If you're *gene positive and starting to experience symptoms*, the future self you've imagined and dreaded for so long begins to take shape; and
- If you're *gene negative*, your identity includes the knowledge that your life is a stark contrast to what it could have been and to the lives of family members who inherited the disease.

Family caregivers also experience changes in identity. First, they transition from traditional roles of parent, child, sibling, partner, or spouse, into an ever-expanding caregiving role. When loved ones pass away, family caregivers must then learn how to live a new life that is no longer shaped by providing care. These changing identities are all tied to something called anticipatory grief, which means experiencing grief in the present for the many things that will eventually be lost to the disease, including the *future-that-could-have-been* if not for Huntington's disease. These changing identities affect not only how members of the HD community think about the future, but also how they approach each day and make important life decisions.

A livable life

When you know that your future will or might include a debilitating neurodegenerative disease, and that the time before symptoms appear gets shorter every day, you must figure out how to approach life in a way that makes the most of what could be a shortened amount of time. Brianna is a young woman from Maryland who made two plans for her life when she was at risk. When she received her positive test result, she knew which one to follow.

No one in Brianna's family knew about Huntington's disease when her parents got married, even though her grandma was already exhibiting early symptoms. Her grandma eventually received an HD diagnosis, and Brianna's mom tested positive soon after that. Brianna has no memories of her grandma before she became bedbound. In old photos, Brianna sees a person she never knew. "There are pictures of her holding me as a baby, and she has the meanest-looking face," Brianna said. "She didn't have control of her face anymore. I have to remind myself that she loved me very much despite what her angry expressions suggested."

When Brianna watched her parents' wedding video a few years ago, she was surprised to see her grandma walking and participating in the festivities. "It was weird to finally see the living person on the other end of the face I saw in pictures," she said. Brianna also noticed her grandma's chorea. As the video continued, Brianna heard her grandma's voice for the first time. "I sobbed like a baby," she said. "She had always been this unobtainable person in my life because I couldn't get to know her through anything other than stories and images."

When Brianna's parents decided to have a baby, they considered conceiving via in vitro fertilization to avoid passing the disease to the next generation. The procedure was new, though, so they didn't feel comfortable pursuing it and chose to conceive naturally. As an only child of busy parents who both have PhDs in chemistry, Brianna felt pressure to do well in school. She developed an eclectic collection of hobbies and even took trapeze classes during summer breaks.

Life felt normal until the summer before Brianna started high school. Her mom was let go from her job because her early HD symptoms were interfering with her ability to perform her work duties, but Brianna hadn't noticed any difference yet. One evening during Brianna's freshman year, her parents asked to talk with her. Brianna settled into her usual spot at the top of the stairs while her parents sat on the couch. Brianna's mom was crying, and her dad told her to come downstairs, which meant this was going to be a serious conversation. Brianna wondered if her mom had cancer because she had gone to the doctor recently.

Brianna was confused when her dad said, "Mom has Huntington's." When Brianna asked what that was, he replied, "What your grandma has." Brianna felt discombobulated. This conversation didn't make sense, so she said, "You knew what was wrong with grandma all along, and nobody thought to tell me?" Brianna had known for a long time that there was something wrong with her grandmother, but no one had ever given it a name. When Brianna's parents told her she had a 50-50 chance of carrying the expanded HD gene, Brianna couldn't believe she couldn't get tested right away. "I was mad that I had to wait until I was 18 to find out something that was life changing for me." That was still four years away.

In the meantime, Brianna began providing some of her mom's care. As her mom's HD symptoms progressed, Brianna found it difficult when other people took notice. "I remember one time I had friends over, and mom burned the mac-and-cheese she made for us. I don't know how you burn mac-and-cheese," she said. When her friends asked about the brown bits, Brianna wanted to save face with her friends, so she told them that was how her mom liked it. Her friends refused to eat it, so Brianna ate the mac-and-cheese and found something else for her friends to eat. "I wanted to cry," she said. "I didn't want to see mom's feelings hurt if no one ate the food she had so kindly prepared for us. I did it for my mom because I love her."

One week after her 18th birthday, Brianna met with a genetic counselor to start the genetic testing process. She wanted to know if she faced the same fate as her mom, or if she would get to live a normal life after being her mom's caregiver. During that initial visit, the doctors asked her several times if she was certain she wanted to know her gene status and if getting tested was the best decision. They even asked if her parents were forcing her to get tested. "I had been waiting so long to know this answer," Brianna said. "I was 100 percent sure I wanted to know. There's nothing they could have told me that day that would have changed my mind, but they tried. The entirety of the day, they kept telling me, 'No, you shouldn't do it. Just wait a couple years to make sure you're certain.'" She was not dissuaded.

Brianna's parents and two of her lifelong friends accompanied her to her final appointment to receive her genetic test result. That morning, she had written in her journal that she was grateful she would have her friends with her. She was nervous about what was to come, but she knew their presence would be calming. Brianna thinks her family and friends had more difficulty coping with her positive test result than she did. Right after her appointment, Brianna wanted to ignore her positive result and sing along to the music in the car, but her friends and family were silent. "It took a while for me to realize they were mourning the future they thought they had with me because they hadn't had to emotionally process that yet," Brianna said. "My mom was mourning the fact that she didn't do IVF when she had the chance. I realized that everybody else was experiencing their own kind of loss, to the point that they weren't able to give me what I wanted and needed at that moment. I didn't want to be sad."

Soon after she received her test result, Brianna attended an HD camp for youth where she was surrounded by others from HD families. Some were at risk, some had tested negative, and some were gene positive like her. "There were a bunch of other people roughly my age who hadn't tested yet, and there were a couple people older than me that had tested," she said. "It was nice to bounce ideas off of each other and build up a community." Brianna continues to build that community through social media groups, where she's found a space to ask questions and share lessons learned. "The internet has brought people together from all over the world to tackle some of the bigger issues and help individuals determine how to best handle situations."

While Brianna knows her childhood friends will always be there for her, she values the additional support she finds when interacting with the HD community. "They are the ones who share your experience, your story," she said. "They understand what you're going through – the pressures of caretaking, the pressures of planning for the future while still so young, and the relationship pressures that can disintegrate marriages for any number of reasons. People outside of the community just don't understand that."

Before Brianna got tested, she made a plan for how she would approach her test result, no matter if it was positive or negative. She developed two distinct plans for her future – the long-term plan in which she was gene negative and free to do whatever she chose, and the short-term plan in which she was gene positive and needed to prepare for HD symptom onset. Knowing her fate helps Brianna plan her future, including how to spend the time between now and when symptoms appear. "I call it my livable life," she said, "where I'm able to do everything I want to do. I consider my livable life up until I'm 50. Logistically, it's probably going to be less, but we aren't going to talk about that." Now that she knows she's gene positive, a PhD program is off the table because she doesn't want to spend that much time in school. Instead, she is pursuing a master's degree in biology where she uses zebrafish to research how diabetes affects growth and movement. She's preparing for a science-based career she will enjoy that will provide enough money to cover future medical costs.

To cope with being gene positive, Brianna stays busy and does her best not to focus on the negative aspects of Huntington's disease. "It's super cliché," she said, "but I try to look for the positives in every moment. It makes it so much more bearable because you learn to accept things the way they are rather than be upset that things didn't turn out the way you wanted." She seeks out adventure and wants to experience as much as she can while she's able. She became a certified scuba diver at age 13 and enjoys her family's annual vacations to the Caribbean. She's even gone paragliding, parasailing, and skydiving to experience all the world has to offer. In college, she joined seven clubs including the quidditch team, the sailing team, and the glassblowing club to meet people and try new things.

Looking ahead, Brianna thinks it will be especially hard when she starts noticing symptoms in herself. "Obviously, there's the sadness of losing out on the extra years that you theoretically could have had," she said, "but do something valuable with the years you're here. Make those impacts now, make those friends. I think being an extrovert has helped because I'm busy all the time – that's probably another coping mechanism. I don't give myself a lot of time to sit and be sad and think about it. I'm going to live my livable life until somebody tells me that my livable life is either shorter or longer than I originally thought. Fifty is a nice average – it's not 100, and it's not zero."

Brianna's mom now lives in an assisted living facility. She fits right in with the other residents. "My mom's always been an old soul at heart," Brianna said. "She started a knitting club. She's so personable, so lively, and so funny. It just takes her a little longer to communicate." Brianna chose to attend a college a few hours away so she could get home easily if needed. It's important to Brianna to maintain a relationship with her mom now that they don't see each other every day. She regularly uploads pictures and messages to a digital wall display in her mom's room. "I try to make sure I do my weekly calls with her, because at a certain point, I'm not going to be able to do that anymore," she said. "It's important that I don't miss out on this time with her."

When Brianna returned home during college breaks, she worked as a receptionist at her mom's assisted living facility. She was able to work there during the COVID-19 pandemic when her college classes were online. As a staff member, she felt lucky to see her mom regularly at a time when most residents were unable to see their families in person. When Brianna was at work, her mom sat nearby. "Even if I wasn't able to talk to her while working," Brianna said, "it still felt like she was part of my day, part of my life, and that made her happy... and I got to spend time with her."

The assisted living facility is often understaffed, so Brianna's mom doesn't always get the level of care Brianna would like to see. "The staff who care for you determines how you look, how you feel – those kinds of things," Brianna said. "I'd never move her unless she told me she's unhappy. I just want them to take care of her like I would." A local HD organization offered to send someone to the facility to provide education on caring for HD patients, but the facility has yet to accept the offer.

Belonging to an HD family has taught Brianna a lot about herself. "I'm a hell of a lot stronger than I used to give myself credit for," she said. "I've been through just about everything that can happen to a person. I think adding HD to my plate didn't feel like that big of a challenge because of all the other things I had already overcome. It's been eye-opening that I can handle a lot of things with power and grace. I still wake up with a smile on my face and still enjoy life for being life – nothing less and nothing more." She also appreciates the people around her. "I find hope in the fact that there are people who like me and enjoy my presence. It means that if I die early, I will be missed; and if I am able to overcome HD in some way, people will be excited I made it."

As Brianna described it, a *livable life* refers to the time before HD symptom onset. This period is important for those who are gene positive or at risk, but it is also important for HD families. During this period, life is unimpeded by the changing physical, cognitive, and behavioral symptoms of Huntington's disease. It is the time to live a full life. For many, this period passes by too quickly; it is precious and should not be wasted.

A *livable life* also refers to how we spend our time and care for our loved ones. Members of the HD community have limited time to make intentional decisions about what they want life to look like, and many want this time to be meaningful. So, people might spend more time with loved ones to create lasting memories, advocate for better care for a loved one with Huntington's disease, focus on personal wellbeing, or become an advocate for the HD community. In this case, a livable life refers to living life with intention and meaning when the future is daunting or uncertain.

Brianna's *livable life* term is meaningful and encompasses many of the ways people approach Huntington's disease, whether they're at risk, gene positive, gene negative, or have family members with the disease. It is a positive affirmation of living life as well as you can and making life for a loved one with Huntington's disease as good as it can be. There is no doubt that being impacted by Huntington's disease comes with many complex challenges and emotions. It would be easy to give up, but that's not what people shared as they told their stories. While people talked about extremely difficult situations, they also talked about the things they do to make the best of a life that includes Huntington's disease – the things they do to create and maintain their own livable life.

When Brianna learned that other people identify with her *livable life* term, she said, "I'm glad others resonate with the ideas and wording I frequently use to remind myself that my life is fantastic, and I need to work with the time I'm blessed with and not worry about how much time I might lose." Interestingly, even though she knows she's gene positive, Brianna still has a dual view of her future. She is currently living her livable life, but her HD life awaits her.

Approaching each day

To cope with belonging to an HD family, I do a lot of emotional processing. My thoughts rarely sit still, so I have an ongoing internal conversation about what's on my mind. I feel better when I actively do something because it gives me some control over my own HD narrative. When I was newly at risk, I learned as much as I could about Huntington's disease and started visiting my brother and his family more often. I attended a support group during the first few years, and I helped start an annual fundraising walk. These actions helped me connect with others and make a positive contribution to the HD community. But there are times when I am overwhelmed by emotions related to how Huntington's disease impacts me and my family. When this happens, I tend to withdraw inward or turn up the music to drown out my thoughts – the louder the better.

HD families face overwhelming worries related to family members' gene status, care decisions, finances, and so much more. Maintaining a livable life requires finding ways to cope with the many challenges of the disease – something that looks different from person to person. It's important to find ways to express concerns, whether that means seeing a therapist, talking with friends or family, connecting with others in the HD community, or keeping a journal. Sometimes, relief can be found through physical activity, artistic expression, or spending time in nature. Some people stay as busy as possible to avoid thinking about Huntington's disease, and some deal with things a little at a time. Others focus on living life as normally as possible to avoid letting Huntington's disease dominate every day. Some even choose to live a spectacular life.

If you're impacted by Huntington's disease and positive coping strategies aren't working, it is crucial to seek help to minimize the risk of turning to harmful coping strategies like alcohol or substance abuse or thinking about suicide. Reach out to family members, friends, a therapist, a faith leader, or an HD organization for help.

Everyone impacted by Huntington's disease must find their own way of coping with what the disease takes away. Finding strategies that work can be challenging, as is maintaining them over time, something Darcy Hawkins knows well. She is close to her family members who have Huntington's disease, and she is gene positive herself. She relies heavily on her faith, and she actively decides every day to have a positive attitude.

Darcy has few memories of her grandfather, but one that stands out is saying goodbye to him at the hospital before he passed away. She was just seven years old, and it would be 25 years before her dad's HD diagnosis would explain that her grandpa had died of Huntington's disease. Darcy's dad remembers seeing a binder at his parents' house long ago that said something about Huntington's disease, but he never looked at it or thought much about it. Darcy's dad was surprised when his brother asked if he wanted to get tested. His brother had known about Huntington's disease for years, but Darcy's dad had not.

The two brothers went through the genetic testing process at the same time. Darcy's uncle received a negative test result, but her dad's positive result explained why he no longer seemed like the person Darcy remembered from her childhood. "He was a fun dad," she said. "He always went to everything – first one to come to your sports, last one to leave. He was the life of the party, my teddy bear, not a mean bone in his body." Now, her dad spends a lot of time watching TV. He's lost weight, acquired a short fuse, and experienced significant cognitive decline. He retired early after his job performance was affected by multiple falls, unsafe driving, and arguing with co-workers. Darcy knows her dad's behavioral changes are caused by the disease, but they are still hard to deal with at times.

Darcy was still learning about Huntington's disease when she decided to get tested just five months after her dad's diagnosis. She was going through a divorce at the time and figured her life couldn't get much worse. "I didn't really process it," she said. "I just kind of did it." When Darcy received a positive result, her first instinct was to make sure everybody else in her family was okay. She was determined to stay strong in the face of her new future.

Darcy didn't realize the magnitude of her own positive result until her younger sister tested negative a year later. As her family rejoiced and talked about all the things her sister could do now – like have children without worry – Darcy realized she would never have that future. In her blog, she wrote, "Although I shared their happiness, I also felt broken for the first time since testing positive." Darcy's older sister tested positive a year after that, and her younger half-brother is at risk. "To say the last five years have been an emotional rollercoaster would be an understatement, but I wouldn't change a single thing," she said.

Now that Darcy knows more about Huntington's disease, she thinks she should have taken more time before getting tested to consider what a test result would mean. It would have been good to have life insurance in place, and she hadn't thought about how receiving her own positive result would impact her dad. "I didn't know it would affect him more, you know? There was a good year that every time I saw him, he'd say he was sorry when we said goodbye," she said. "That was tough."

Symptom onset can have a significant impact on relationships. Darcy's dad was around 40 years old and going through a divorce when his HD symptoms began. Darcy's gene-positive sister also divorced around the time of her symptom onset. "They were both married for approximately 20 years, and it seemed to be right around the time of their divorces when things started to crumble," Darcy said.

Darcy sees changes in her dad that people outside the family don't see. He's still able to walk, but he has changed mentally, and Darcy knows things will continue to change. "My dad and my sister are my best friends," she said. "It seems like every year gets harder. When one of them can't meet me at a restaurant and have dinner – I think some of those changes will be hard; and then, I guess, whenever I feel symptoms in myself."

There are parts of Darcy's story that she doesn't often share but wishes she could. "I don't talk much about kids, mostly because I'm almost 40," she said. "I've been married and divorced, and being a mom is all I ever wanted." Dating has been challenging because, as Darcy says, "Who wants to gamble on me?" She's always been up front about her gene status because she doesn't want to be in a relationship with anyone who is unwilling to travel that path with her. Darcy has been dating her new boyfriend for several months. He's very supportive and makes her feel seen and special. "I'm hopeful now," she said. "I try to protect other people. Sometimes, you care so much about someone that you don't want them to be by your side and have to take care of you. I think like that from time to time, and that probably has to do with protecting my heart. I'm learning to let go and let people make their own decision instead of doing that for them."

Darcy copes by getting involved. She's active in the HD community and has received awards for her work. She serves on the Minnesota

HDSA board, speaks at events, has an online blog, participates in research studies, and is involved in HDSA's National Youth Alliance and other youth-centered programs. She's passionate about helping young people think through all angles of the genetic testing process so they can make an informed decision. Darcy finds support through her church and at a monthly HDSA support group. She especially appreciates spending time with her support group's social worker, Jessica, who understands the disease and is comforting. Darcy and Jessica's relationship extends beyond Huntington's disease; they can talk about anything.

To cope with having Huntington's disease in her life, Darcy stays busy and does her best to maintain a positive outlook, but it takes constant effort. "At first, I forced myself to believe that I was going to be okay," she said. "I basically lied to myself until I believed it. It eventually became natural to think like that. You have to make the decision every single day. Some days are going to be bad, and that's okay. You just have to make the decision to be happy over and over again." Darcy counts her blessings often. "I have a lot of faith in what God has in store for me. I'm not sure there will be a cure in my lifetime, but I'm hopeful in everyday things. You don't have to let this define you. You can still live a full life. HD has given me so much more than it will ever take away. My family's always been close, but we definitely have a deeper appreciation of smaller things. It's given me a good community and good friends, and I have a passion for living a good life, not just living."

Important life decisions

Huntington's disease adds a complicated layer to making important life decisions, especially choosing a career, entering into romantic relationships, and having children. If I had known about Huntington's disease when my dad was still alive, I would have been in my teens and 20s rather than in my 40s when I started living life in preparation for the

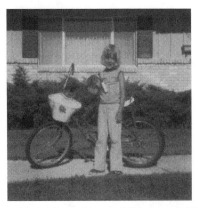

I was able to dream big as a kid because I didn't know I needed to take Huntington's disease into account when making major life decisions.

possibility of having a neurodegenerative disease. I might not have taken the time to pursue a graduate degree. I might have hesitated to have a romantic relationship or consider marriage knowing that I might need my partner to be my caregiver one day. I might not have had kids for fear of passing on the disease or raising children within an HD family. Even though I worried that I might one day have the same thing my dad did, I knew nothing about Huntington's disease. I had no clue what his symptoms meant for my future, so I made these important life decisions freely – just like most people.

These decisions look very different when you factor in Huntington's disease. When young people in the HD community consider what they want their adult life to look like, they ask themselves questions like: Is it worth investing time in training for the job or career I want? Will I be able to complete my training and pay off student loans in time to save money for future medical costs? Will I be able to perform the job duties of my chosen career if I start having symptoms? Should I choose a career that interests me or one that helps the HD community? Due to the possibility of limited time, there might be only one chance to make the right decision. The intensity of these decisions goes far beyond what most young people face.

Romantic relationships are especially challenging for people who are at risk or gene positive. Dating requires figuring out the right time to tell someone about Huntington's disease. The consensus is not too soon, and not too late, which is impossible to pinpoint. It's common to worry about being rejected once a potential partner learns about Huntington's disease or becoming a burden one day to the person you love most. Many people tell their partner that they do not have to stay in the relationship because of how hard it is to belong to an HD family. It can be hard to accept that someone would willingly take on the burden of becoming your caregiver, so some people avoid becoming close or intimate altogether.

When deciding whether to have children, top concerns include the possibility of passing the disease to the next generation and having children who will grow up witnessing the decline of a gene-positive parent. Those who decide to have children can take advantage of family planning options that use genetic testing to ensure children will not inherit the expanded gene. These options can be expensive and invasive, however, making it difficult for some families to access them. Couples may choose to have children naturally and hope a cure is found before children who inherit Huntington's disease become symptomatic. Or couples can adopt, although some adoption agencies do not allow a prospective parent to adopt if they are at risk or gene positive. Having a family is important to Angela, a gene-positive young woman from Brisbane, Australia. She was young when she got married, and she and her husband took advantage of in vitro fertilization and genetic testing to have an HD-free child. She is grateful that she can maximize her time with her young family before her symptoms begin.

Growing up, Angela heard stories about *something in the family* that affected family members both physically and mentally. "They had no idea what it was," she said. "They just knew that people got very sick, and they had only a couple of years to live after that." HD symptoms can look different from person to person, even within the same family. This was true in Angela's family. Her grandpa's sister had physical and cognitive symptoms that were initially misdiagnosed as Parkinson's disease. Her grandpa's brother had violent outbursts and would disappear for a week at a time, returning injured and out of money. He couldn't always remember what had happened while he was away. When her grandpa's brother was eventually diagnosed with Huntington's disease, Angela said, "it finally gave my family clarity. That was a big turning point in my family." Angela's grandpa and his sister were both later diagnosed with Huntington's disease as well.

When Angela was a young girl, she thought her grandpa was strange and different. He had special cutlery and cups for eating and drinking. He also had unusual hand movements and couldn't sit still in his chair. In the later stages of his disease, her grandpa had speech difficulties and became forgetful. Soon after Angela's grandpa died, her mom started having chorea in her hands. Angela's mom never had a genetic test, so her HD diagnosis was based on symptoms and family history. Her primary symptoms included depression, poor decision-making, extreme mood swings, forgetfulness, trouble swallowing, and chorea.

Angela grew up in a small city in Australia, so her mom had to travel to HD appointments by airplane. When her mom's symptoms progressed to the point that she was no longer able to fly, she had to stop seeing her HD doctor. Angela's parents eventually separated, so Angela helped her brother, aunt, and uncle care for her mom until her mom moved to an assisted living facility. Her mom later became bedbound and nearly unable to communicate. She died of Huntington's disease at the age of 57.

Angela knew from an early age that she wanted to get tested when she turned 18 because she wanted to know how to approach decisions related to career goals, having children, and finances. Angela had always been told she was like her dad and his family, so she was certain she was gene negative. Angela was stunned when she received a positive test result. "I still remember that moment so vividly," she said. "My whole body went numb, and the room fell completely silent. I couldn't look at my dad or my boyfriend. I froze. My mind instantly began rushing with endless thoughts of what my life will be like." She became physically ill after that appointment and went to the emergency room later that day where she learned she was in shock.

Coping with her positive result was difficult, especially during the first few weeks. Support from friends and family helped, as did attending support groups and developing stronger ties with the staff at her local HD charity. Angela also copes by setting three major goals for herself each year and being involved in the HD community. She is an HDYO ambassador and a member of HD-CAB. She speaks publicly about Huntington's disease, and she recently volunteered as a board member for her local state HD charity. In this role, she participated in the process of combining all of Australia's state HD charities under a single umbrella organization called Huntington's Australia.

Angela felt very alone when she first tested positive, even though she had her family's support. She wanted to connect with other young adults to talk about life decisions she'd have to make, including family planning. She couldn't find other young people in her small town who had gone through predictive genetic testing, so she widened her search to her state and then all of Australia and beyond. She spent hours searching online and found countless websites and support groups in the United Kingdom and the United States but nothing on her side of the world. She also found that most resources and support groups focused on people who are family caregivers or symptomatic, not people like her who are gene positive but presymptomatic.

Angela was determined to give a voice to the next generation of Australians who are at risk or presymptomatic, so she turned her focus to creating opportunities to support HD youth in her country. She worked with others to create resources, and her local state HD charity even held a youth camp. After attending the HDYO Congress in Scotland, Angela and a friend created a Facebook group to connect HD youth across Australia. It continues to grow.

After Angela tested positive for Huntington's disease, she gave her boyfriend the option of leaving, but he didn't. They married in the fall of 2020 and met with a fertility specialist a few months later. Angela always wanted to have kids, but only if she could ensure they wouldn't inherit Huntington's disease. Being gene positive means her chances of adopting in Australia are low, so she and her husband chose to conceive through a process called in vitro fertilization with pre-implantation genetic diagnosis (IVF with PGD). In this procedure, fertilized embryos are tested for Huntington's disease, and only those that are gene negative are implanted during the IVF process. Angela started an Instagram page to document her journey with Huntington's disease and IVF. Sharing her story raises awareness and helps her connect with others facing similar situations. "Social media is good for making those connections," she said, "especially in Australia and internationally, and especially for Huntington's."

In Angela's first round of IVF, 20 eggs were retrieved but only three were successfully fertilized, and none could be used for a transfer. Angela and her husband took a break for several months to save more money. Even though Australia's Medicare program now covers some of the cost of genetic testing, the remaining out-of-pocket cost for each round of IVF egg retrieval is around $8,000-$10,000 AUD. Angela and her husband also paused to give themselves time to focus on their mental health before starting a second round. The second round was successful: 25 eggs were retrieved, six were sent for genetic testing, and three were viable for transfer. Angela remembers her first ultrasound after the IVF transfer was successful. "She was a little tiny thing on the screen, like the size of a small bean," Angela said. "As soon as we heard the heartbeat, we were like, okay, that makes it more surreal. This is going to happen." The young parents now have a healthy, HD-free, baby girl.

Angela and her husband still have two HD-free frozen embryos, so they have two chances to have a second child. They decided early in the IVF process that if neither of those attempts results in a pregnancy, they won't go through another round of egg harvesting because the procedure is difficult and expensive. Making this decision long before the situation arises reduces Angela's stress. She knows that having kids when she is young extends the number of good years she can spend with her family. Angela is about 10 years younger than her mom was when Angela was born. "That 10 years is going to be a big thing," she said. "I was in year seven – so primary school here in Australia – when my mum became symptomatic. That's not going to be the case for my daughter. She might be a freshman in high school, or hopefully have all her schooling completed before I become very symptomatic. That's going to be a huge difference."

Angela has faced criticism from family, strangers, and even some in the HD community for having her daughter. "Some people have said how cruel it is to bring a baby into the world when she's going to have a parent who is sick. A few people even called me selfish because my child might feel pressured into being a caregiver for me when I'm older," Angela said. "People randomly pass away all the time. I've had many family members pass away from cancer. Some people focus so much on the HD that they forget all these other things that can happen. Being realistic, every day is a risk; every day is a blessing. I'm trying not to take those comments to heart, but at the same time, they do affect me."

When critics are from the HD community, Angela finds it especially disheartening. "If they've been a carer for someone with HD, they know what it's like. For me to still want children," she said, "that shouldn't be a complete no. I've gone through the effort. I've gone through the full IVF journey. For someone to say, 'You shouldn't have done that; you shouldn't have had kids.' If anything, I'm doing something beneficial. I'm breaking the Huntington's cycle instead of having kids naturally." Angela knows people are entitled to their opinions, but she doesn't have to agree with them.

Thinking ahead, Angela thinks it's important to have a plan in place for talking to her daughter about Huntington's disease long before it's needed. When her grandpa started having HD symptoms, Angela's parents used a children's book to help her understand her grandpa's disease. They waited until she was older to tell her about the genetic component, something Angela will never have to worry about for her daughter. "Hubby and I spoke recently about how we're going to introduce HD to her and explain that at some point I'm going to be sick," she said. "I've still got the book to explain HD to kids. It says elderly people in this family get weird movements; they go through mood swings. It explains some of the common symptoms of HD so it's easy for them to understand. It'll be a nice book to easily guide her through it. I've got photos and videos of my mum as well, so when my daughter's older, I can show her those."

Being a young mom gives Angela a new perspective on memories of her own mom. "They were always precious memories," Angela said. "But now I see them from a different perspective. Until you become a mom yourself, I don't think you can see that. I was thinking of a memory just the other day. We went to the lake and went fishing. Mum was truly symptomatic at this stage, but she was smiling. She liked the beach. Those kinds of memories are extra special."

Knowing her daughter will not have Huntington's disease makes being a new mom very poignant. "I know my daughter is never going to have to worry about it," Angela said. "She's going to have good health as far as we know. All of that is not a worry. At some point in the future, though, I'm going to become symptomatic. I was 22 when my mom passed. Hopefully, my daughter's going to be older." Angela also thinks about what her mom is missing. "She knew I was engaged, but she didn't get to see me get married or be there for the birth of Bub. She's never going to watch her grow up. It's that kind of bittersweet thing."

Angela plans to pay close attention to new memories she's making with her young family. "Since testing gene positive," she said, "HD has changed my view on life. I'm now able to see a hopeful aspect in almost every situation. Despite the negativity it may bring to a person's life, I always look for the positive aspect in any situation and the memorable moments to cherish and reflect back on. I know that I've been incredibly lucky to have the option to be tested and plan for the future." Angela is actively creating a life that is meaningful to her – a life in which she can be a mother to a daughter who will never have Huntington's disease.

When I first learned we are an HD family, I thought if I was gene positive, I wouldn't be able to choose my own direction once symptoms appeared. I thought my HD future would be set in stone. What I've learned from my conversations, though, is that there is a lot of room in a life with Huntington's disease to make choices. Decisions can be made to maximize quality of life, and it is possible to develop an attitude and an outlook on life that helps cope with the many difficulties of the disease. There is nothing easy about a life with Huntington's disease, but it is possible to have a livable life all the same.

I think a lot about what it means to me to have a livable life. I'm grateful I can continue to be an active participant in the lives of my husband and kids, and they can continue to know me as my true self. Small moments of being comfortable together with people I care about carry more meaning than they once did and have become a cornerstone of my livable life. I appreciate my very ordinary life. For my brother, things like eating pizza, watching his favorite sports teams play, and spending time with his family make him happy. He also has a nonfamily caregiver who genuinely cares about his wellbeing. These are some of the things that make his life as livable as it can be.

The HD community faces immense challenges, but there are meaningful changes that could make possible a more livable life for those impacted by Huntington's disease. First would be more awareness. Increased familiarity with Huntington's disease and its symptoms could lead to more acceptance and fewer misunderstandings about what is causing a person's movements or behaviors. If doctors and nonfamily caregivers better understood the disease and its impact on families, they could provide earlier, more appropriate, and higher-quality care. If policymakers understood the challenges HD families face perhaps there would be more support for legislation to address HD families' healthcare needs and provide timely access to much-needed federal benefits.

Another meaningful change would be increased research funding from government agencies, private foundations, and pharmaceuticals. More funds are needed to reach the HD community's goal of finding treatments as soon as possible to slow, halt, or prevent disease progression. In the meantime, the HD community would benefit from filling gaps in services, especially in rural areas with little access to HD resources and in countries where there is little understanding of

Huntington's disease. The JHD community would also benefit from more support, more education, and more opportunities to connect with each other. While the HD community has advocates working on each of these issues, these continue to be areas of great need – areas where there is work to be done to move toward a more livable life for the HD community.

GENETIC TESTING

Being at risk for Huntington's disease and thinking about whether to go through the predictive genetic testing process was one of the most intense and stressful experiences I've had. The fact that a genetic test exists added weight to my HD experience. Testing dominated my thoughts the entire time I was at risk, and the testing decision felt monumental and far from straightforward. Right after my brother's diagnosis, I initially thought I should get tested so I could know what was coming and plan accordingly. It didn't take long, though, to realize there were pros and cons to consider, and I needed time to make the decision that was right for me. Finding out my gene status would be easy – the answer could be revealed by a simple blood test – but did I truly want to know if my life would be altered by a neurodegenerative disease? Would my life be better or worse if I knew that answer? And how would I cope if I tested positive?

When going through the genetic testing process, there is no way to predict what the result will be, how you will react, and how your life will change once your gene status is revealed, no matter how much thought you put into it. It's an emotionally challenging experience every step of the way. Getting tested means having to cope with a test result, whether it's positive, negative, or in the gray area. Deciding to remain at risk means having to cope with the continued uncertainty of an unknown gene status. Outside the HD community, there is little understanding of the complexity of this decision and plenty of curiosity about why most people who are at risk choose not to get tested.

Genetic testing basics

A simple blood test for Huntington's disease became available soon after the 1993 discovery of the single gene that determines HD gene status. Only recent generations have had the ability to know their gene status before symptom onset and take advantage of genetic testing to have children without passing on the disease. Before this discovery, researchers thought most people at risk for Huntington's disease would want to get tested if given the chance. Now that a test is available, however, only a small percentage of at-risk people do so. The exact percentage is unknown, but estimates range from 3 to 25 percent. There is currently no cure or disease-modifying treatment for Huntington's disease, so there is no medical benefit to knowing your gene status. If therapies become available to prevent or alter disease progression before symptoms appear, at-risk individuals may be more likely to get tested.

The development of a simple blood test for Huntington's disease opened the door to a variety of genetic testing options. *Diagnostic genetic testing* can rule out or confirm a suspected HD diagnosis if a clinical examination points to Huntington's disease and other diseases have been excluded. A known family history of the disease is not required. A doctor typically looks for chorea – the motor symptom of Huntington's disease – before making a clinical diagnosis of disease onset. Guidelines set forth by HDSA recommend that children under age 18 should only undergo genetic testing if they show symptoms that are consistent with Juvenile Huntington's disease and cannot be attributed to another disease or disorder.

HDSA guidelines recommend genetic counseling for anyone who seeks out *predictive genetic testing*, a process that allows someone to learn their HD gene status in the absence of symptoms. An individual's decision to get tested should not be influenced by others – not even family members or medical professionals – and testing should take place within a supportive environment and when life stressors are minimal. The testing process should not be rushed and should give the patient enough time to be certain of their decision. Patients retain the right to stop or postpone the process at any time. Genetic counselors should advise patients of potential adverse emotional responses to their test result and offer additional counseling after the result appointment. Patients should be aware that a positive test result can reveal the gene status of family members who may wish to remain at risk, such as a parent or identical twin. A genetic counselor can help navigate complex situations like these.

Several genetic testing options allow people who are at risk or gene positive to have children without passing on the disease. *Prenatal genetic testing* of a fetus can be done during pregnancy via chorionic villus sampling or amniocentesis. If testing reveals a fetus is gene positive, parents can decide to terminate the pregnancy if abortion is an available option where they live. If a parent is at risk, then a positive test for the fetus reveals that the parent is gene positive as well. In this case, couples are faced with deciding whether to terminate a pregnancy at the same time that they learn one of them is gene positive.

If an at-risk parent does not want to know their own HD status, they can take advantage of a method called *exclusion testing*. In this method, a section of the fetus's DNA that includes the HD gene is compared to the same section of DNA from both of its parents and from one of the parents of the at-risk parent. This method is not as precise as prenatal genetic testing and does not indicate if a fetus is gene positive or gene negative, nor does it indicate the gene status of the at-risk parent. Instead, exclusion testing indicates whether a fetus's chance of having inherited the expanded HD gene is low or 50-50. Parents can then decide whether to continue or terminate the pregnancy.

Another option for having an HD-free baby is *in vitro fertilization with pre-implantation genetic diagnosis* (IVF with PGD). In this procedure, fertilized embryos are tested for Huntington's disease, and only those that are gene negative are implanted during the IVF process. In this procedure, an at-risk parent can ask not to be informed of the gene status of un-implanted embryos, thus concealing their own HD gene status. IVF with PGD is expensive and not always covered by health insurance. It is also an exhausting process that is not always successful. Some couples go through multiple rounds of IVF before becoming pregnant.

Other options for having an HD-free baby include adoption or using donated eggs, sperm, or embryos that do not carry the expanded gene.

Living at risk

Before I got tested for Huntington's disease, people around me were curious about my choice to remain at risk. Some were puzzled that I would willingly choose not to know if I was going to develop Huntington's disease someday, while others didn't think they could go through the testing process themselves. I have found that people outside the HD community are captivated by and love to discuss the possibility of knowing what the future holds. Many people share what they think they would do in the same situation without understanding the complex feelings and experiences that may be attached to this decision. When it's not your reality, it's a fascinating thought exercise.

When I was at risk, I was on high alert for clues that might indicate I was exhibiting HD symptoms. My thoughts quickly turned to Huntington's disease if I stumbled, dropped an item, or forgot something. It was easy to feel like I was under a microscope as I wondered what my family noticed. I worried they might see signs I didn't. This constant watching and being-watched was nerve wracking and amplified my worries about possibly having Huntington's disease.

I was never 100 percent certain that the symptoms I thought I noticed meant I was gene positive, but many at-risk people do reach that conclusion. It's a constant mind game regardless.

When you are at risk, it is natural to compare yourself to HD family members and assume similarities in personality or appearance mean that you also inherited the expanded HD gene. In my family, only males have had the disease in recent generations – my brother, my dad, and my grandpa. It would be easy to think the odds were in my favor because I'm female, but that had no bearing on my own 50-50 risk. It would also be easy to assume that if one sibling tests positive, another will test negative, but again, each sibling has their own 50-50 risk of inheriting Huntington's disease.

There are many reasons people choose to remain at risk. Many people worry about how they would cope with a positive result. How would they face the years before and after symptom onset? Would they lose all hope for the future or regret testing once they knew their result? Would their HD parent feel guilty for passing on Huntington's disease? Some people choose to remain at risk even if they notice HD symptoms because they want to hold onto a future in which having Huntington's disease is still not certain. While remaining at risk is challenging, it allows people to approach their risk on their own terms.

Not everyone thinks about their at-risk status in the same way. Some people have trouble coping with feelings of anxiety and depression related to being at risk, while others remain at risk because they feel receiving a gene-positive result would cause too much emotional burden. Still others feel like everyone is at risk for something, and this is no different. For me, not knowing my gene status fell somewhere on the spectrum between my worst and best possible outcomes. Not knowing offered more possibilities and hope for my future than I thought I would have if I knew for certain I was going to develop Huntington's disease.

Some people choose to remain at risk because they want to focus on the present. Megan chooses to remain at risk because she wants to enjoy her life while things are going well. She grew up as an only child in rural North Dakota, and she was finishing her master's degree in speech language pathology when we spoke. Megan's family had no known history of Huntington's disease, so her dad was misdiagnosed with a variety of mental health disorders before receiving an HD diagnosis when Megan was nine years old.

Her dad's symptoms started before she was born, so Megan doesn't think she ever got to know her *real* dad. She remembers him as an avid outdoorsman who liked home improvement projects and tinkering in the garage. "He was a kid at heart, and he would always play soccer or baseball or hockey – anything we could do outside together," she said. "He enjoyed having fun and spending time with family." Megan's dad worked as an electrician and owned his own business. When he started falling off ladders, forgetting things, and crossing wires on occasion, Megan's mom received calls from clients who thought he was drinking on the job.

Then, Megan's dad started exhibiting aggressive behaviors that were particularly hard to cope with. When Megan was eight, she and her mom moved out of the house temporarily. "Before he was diagnosed and properly medicated, his mood swings were so extreme and unpredictable," Megan said. "It was so hard to understand why he was reacting that way. There's a lot from that year I don't remember, and that's probably my brain keeping myself safe from something I didn't need to experience at eight-and-a-half or nine years old."

She clearly remembers one incident from that time. Megan and her mom returned to the house to get a sleeping bag for a sleepover, and Megan went into the house by herself. "The house was so disheveled, and the dishes were everywhere," Megan said. "He was a very organized person, and I knew that something wasn't right. This wasn't my dad. He was helping me pack up, and he started crying. He broke down and said, 'I feel like I'm losing my mind, and I can't figure out why.'" Megan thinks her dad was relieved when he was diagnosed with Huntington's disease because he had come to believe he was insane. His diagnosis finally explained his symptoms. "After he received that diagnosis," Megan said, "I remember him saying, 'I'm not going crazy. There is something wrong with my brain.' I can't imagine how isolating it must feel to not understand what's happening to your body and your brain."

Megan's dad remained at home for about two years after his diagnosis. During that time, Megan was only left alone with her dad for short periods of time, but it still made her anxious. "I was so nervous he was going to fall or hit his head or lash out," she said. "HD patients are so unpredictable." Megan knows if she had shared her concern with her mom, her mom would have left her alone with him less often, but she didn't want to place more burden on her mom. "It was such a strange role reversal so early in my life," Megan said. "I was a child cutting up my dad's waffles. Four or five years earlier, that's something he did for me."

One morning soon after Megan started sixth grade, she made breakfast for her dad after her mom left for work and before her grandma arrived. "I didn't put enough syrup on his pancakes, and he started choking in front of me," Megan said. "It was the scariest moment of my life. I thought he was going to pass right in front of me. I called my neighbor, who was a nurse, and she came over and helped us. That afternoon, he went into a nursing home." Her dad's first nursing home was an hour away. When his aggression became too much for that nursing home to handle, he was moved to a nursing home two hours away. "Every weekend for four or five years, we spent two hours, three hours, four hours in the car to go visit my dad in a nursing home," she said. "That's not what a typical middle-schooler does on the weekends."

Megan's parents didn't know they needed to plan financially before her dad was diagnosed. The two-year waiting period to get Medicare after her dad qualified for Social Security disability benefits added to the family's financial burden. They had to sell their house and spend half of their retirement savings and much of Megan's college savings to pay the medical bills. Megan's family paid the nursing home bills out-of-pocket for months while they waited. "Even after he passed," Megan said, "we were still dealing with the medical bills and the funeral expenses and all of the things that come with Huntington's and losing your loved one."

While Megan and her mom talk openly about many aspects of Huntington's disease, they don't talk about genetic testing. Megan doesn't want to overburden her mom. She doesn't plan to get tested anytime soon, but it's something she thinks about often. "After I finish school, what's the timeline? Do I want to test? Do I not want to test? That's not something I want to necessarily share with my mom because I feel she has so much guilt and anxiety about that part of this journey," Megan said. "I don't want to fill her in on how I'm feeling until I have a more concrete understanding of what I want to do."

Before getting tested, Megan wants to learn more about long-term care insurance and disability benefits, things most 23-year-olds don't think about. She also wants to figure out how to prepare people close to her for the testing process, especially her mom and her boyfriend of seven years. "There are other people who are part of this journey," she said. "It's not just my decision; it affects them as well."

When Megan tells people about Huntington's disease, she's happy to answer their questions unless they ask if she's been tested – that question is much too personal. She tries to help others understand her point of view by using cancer as an example: "If you knew that 15 years from now, you were going to get cancer and you were going to die, and you weren't going to be able to communicate with your family... I try to get them to understand that if I test, that is essentially what I'm signing up for," she said. "I sign up for knowing my fate, and it's almost like a countdown. I don't know if that's something I want. I want people to understand that even though their question comes from a place of curiosity, it can be a personal and very protected topic."

Megan appreciates having multiple perspectives in her life, including the perspective of a good friend who did not grow up in an HD family. This friend encourages Megan to think about where she is in her life right now. "My life has been kind of crazy," Megan said. "But now I'm at that point where I'm kind of secure and have found my own happiness. My friend said, 'Why would you want to address testing at a time that you're enjoying your life?' And so, for now, I'm not planning on anything. I don't feel that it's a time in my life where I need to know. It's not something that occupies my mind every day, but it's something that's in the back of my mind."

As a college student, Megan is often asked about her 10-year plan. "I despise that question so much," she said. "Ten years from now, I don't know what my life's going to look like. It's overwhelming. I don't have the ability to make a plan without thinking about how Huntington's affects my life. There are logistical things I have to think about. If I'm going to tell you what I want to do in 10 years, then I have to acknowledge the fact that I might have to test for HD, or I might be gene negative, or I might be gene positive. It's such a loaded question. Other people my age don't have to think about long-term care benefits and health insurance, or the impact that this has on their life and their career. It's a question that always kind of stings."

Instead of having a 10-year plan, Megan pinpointed career and life goals she'd like to work toward. This approach removes a lot of pressure. "I want to help HD families through advocacy," she said. "Through my career choice, I want to help clients of all ages communicate with their families better. I think the uncertainty that comes with being in an HD family gives a cautionary approach to everything. I think a lot of us in HD families don't want to make plans because, as we've experienced, plans don't happen the way they should, and people get sick."

Growing up in a small town made it hard to connect with others in the HD community. The nearest HD support group was hours away, and when Megan did attend, very little of what she heard applied to her. No one was her age. Connecting with the HD community online didn't become available until after her dad died. Instead, Megan found support from friends she met at an HDSA convention. "All of us are roughly the same age, and all our dads had Huntington's," she said. "Some of our dads are still living, and some have passed. It was so reassuring to find people who understand how much this experience impacts your everyday life."

Megan's boyfriend is supportive, even though he may not completely understand Huntington's disease. From the beginning of their relationship, Megan's been transparent about how her at-risk status could affect their future together. She told him, "I might be completely dependent on you at some point, and you might have to take care of all the finances and the house. You might have to put me in a nursing home, and all these things that you don't want to have to think about in a relationship." Megan thinks it's hard for her and her at-risk friends to accept that someone would voluntarily share a future with them. "He's chosen to stay in the relationship with me, and that's such an unconditional act of love," she said. "I know I would do it for him in a heartbeat, but it's hard to accept that somebody else would take that on."

Megan has advocated for the HD community since before her dad died. Every May, during HD awareness month, she shares her story with local news outlets. She also shares her story openly in her professional life. "There's a possibility of discrimination," she said, "but I think it is such a small, miniscule problem compared to the importance of giving others a voice, and sharing my experiences, and bringing that connection that I longed for when I was going through my Huntington's disease experience with my dad. It's a part of who I am. I'm okay with whatever may happen in the future because of my advocacy."

As Megan's family has experienced different aspects of Huntington's disease, her outlook on life, her perspectives on Huntington's disease, and her ability to find hope have changed. "I want other people to know that when I was in the thick of our Huntington's disease journey – when my dad was sick – it was tough and depressing," she said. "I think it's reassuring to hear that there is happiness in a life that has Huntington's in it, and just because you have this diagnosis in your family doesn't mean that you're not ever going to be happy. You'll find things that bring you joy and give you hope for the future. I find hope in other people's experiences and the strength that they share through those experiences."

Megan's dad died just after her 15th birthday. She'll always be grateful for the time she got to spend with him after his diagnosis. She cried softly as she said, "I lost him so early in life. There are a lot of things that he didn't get to see me do like high school graduation, prom pictures, college graduation, my master's graduation. He never got to meet my boyfriend. He'll never get to go to my wedding." When Megan was little, her dad often replied to her requests with, "You got it, Chief." For Christmas one year, Megan's mom gave her the wedding band her dad used to wear with that phrase engraved on it. "I get to carry a piece of him with me," Megan said. "It's sweet and reassuring, and I know he's gotten me through a lot of hard things. It's just nice."

The genetic testing decision

The genetic testing decision came up in almost every conversation I had with the HD community, but conversations differed based on where each person was on their testing journey. Each person had their own list of pros and cons, and decisions were affected by how long they had known about their risk, the severity of family members' symptoms, their HD parent's age at symptom onset, and their own personal feelings about testing.

For anyone who is thinking about predictive genetic testing, it is important to understand why you want to know your gene status and consider what will be gained or lost by knowing that answer. It is also important to think about the right time to get tested. Feelings about testing can change over time or as life circumstances change. By the time an at-risk person is old enough to be eligible for testing – which is typically at age 18 – they may have had years to think about what they want to do. A child who decides at age 13 that they want to get tested when they are old enough may or may not change their mind by the time they reach that age. More than one *Livable Lives* storyteller began the testing process but paused before receiving their result. Their answer is still waiting for them if they decide they want to begin again.

Researchers have found that the most common reasons people choose to go through the predictive genetic testing process are to reduce uncertainty and plan for the future. Other common reasons are to provide information to relatives, inform reproductive decision making, and be eligible to participate in clinical trials. When considering predictive genetic testing, it is important to honestly assess how remaining at risk or getting tested would affect your ability to live the life you want to live. Would getting tested ease or increase your anxiety? Are you comfortable with the uncertainty of being at risk, or do you need to know your gene status to make important decisions? The testing decision should be given the time and thought it deserves, and a genetic counselor can help weigh the pros and cons.

Making the decision that maximizes happiness and emotional wellbeing – whether that means remaining at risk, waiting until the right time, or going ahead with testing – should be the priority. Each of these choices takes courage. I got tested to give my kids a chance to have a future free from the uncertainty of being at risk, but not until I was ready to know the answer for myself.

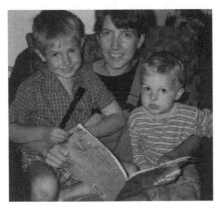

I chose to get tested for my kids.

The genetic testing process

More than four years after I learned I was at risk for Huntington's disease, my own genetic testing process was set in motion when I called to make an appointment with a genetic counselor. It took me several weeks to gather the courage to make that call because it marked a major turning point in my life. I was stepping away from my comfort with not knowing my gene status and into a new life where I would no longer have to wonder if I carried the expanded HD gene. I would finally know my way forward.

I had an initial phone appointment with the genetic counselor to discuss why I wanted to get tested and determine if it made sense to proceed. I then had a brief in-person genetic counseling session before getting my blood drawn. Several weeks later, my husband and I met with the genetic counselor to get my result. The last moments before learning if I was gene positive or negative were a strange mix of anticipation and dread. Was I ready? Once I knew the answer, there would be no going back. It was terrifying.

My testing experience was a scaled-down version of what is outlined in HDSA's protocol for predictive genetic testing. The recommended process varies from country to country, with a longer process in the United Kingdom, for example. HDSA's recommended process includes an initial phone conversation with a genetic counselor plus two in-person appointments. During the first in-person appointment, a genetic counselor reviews the patient's family history and provides an overview of genetics and the genetic testing process. The counselor helps the patient weigh the psychological and social risks of getting tested against the benefits the patient hopes testing will provide. The counselor also assesses whether the patient is emotionally ready to pursue testing. In some cases, this visit includes an optional neurological exam. Finally, a patient's blood is drawn for the genetic test itself.

A patient receives their test result at the second in-person appointment, unless they decide to postpone or cancel. Patients retain the right to withdraw from the process at any time. It is important to have a support person during genetic counseling appointments, especially the result appointment, and a good choice is someone who can provide support without requiring support in return. Some people choose not to take the person they're closest to, so they don't have to cope with that person's reaction on top of their own immediate response. A follow-up phone call or in-person visit can be scheduled with the genetic counselor for several weeks later, and post-test support should be tailored to the needs of the patient. HDSA guidelines don't specify a length of time for the genetic testing process, but research suggests people who receive a test result after a quick process may have more difficulty coping than those who complete a longer process.

Ideally, people getting tested for Huntington's disease would test at a clinic that specializes in Huntington's disease or genetics, and they would work with a neurologist and/or genetic counselor. Not everyone has this type of experience, though, either because they don't have access to these services, or they don't know about them. Barriers to getting tested can include having to travel long distances to meet with a genetic counselor or having to pay out-of-pocket if health insurance doesn't cover predictive genetic testing. In addition, not all genetic counselors are comfortable testing young adults for Huntington's disease. Several *Livable Lives* storytellers faced resistance when their doctor or genetic counselor thought they were too young to learn their gene status, even though they met the age eligibility criteria. Rather than having a conversation about the pros and cons of testing, they felt like their doctor or genetic counselor discouraged them from proceeding. These conversations were often described as a particularly challenging part of the testing process.

Some people want to test anonymously or keep their test result out of their medical record. This can be done by paying for testing out-of-pocket or using a pseudonym. However, testing anonymously could require getting tested again if there is ever a need to show proof of gene status for insurance purposes, to access other benefits, or to participate in a clinical trial. It is important to know that if you test anonymously and later lie about your gene status on paperwork to obtain insurance, you are committing insurance fraud.

HDSA guidelines also recommend investigating options for obtaining life, disability, and long-term care insurance before getting tested. In the United States, these types of insurance are not protected by federal law, so a positive test result could potentially prevent someone from obtaining these insurance benefits. Before my brother was officially diagnosed, his doctor urged him to tell his siblings to obtain life and long-term care insurance. I was late to dinner on my birthday that summer because I was signing paperwork to purchase a long-term care insurance policy. I already had life insurance, but I wanted to cover my bases for addressing future medical costs if I developed Huntington's disease.

My financial advisor was aware of my brother's situation and had consulted with his state-level superiors to make sure I could buy a policy without committing insurance fraud. I had to be able to answer, "no," to the question, "Do you have a parent or sibling with Huntington's disease?" While my brother's MRI and the neurologist's clinical examination pointed to Huntington's disease, he hadn't yet had his blood drawn for a genetic test to confirm his diagnosis. For the time being, my financial advisor and his superiors agreed that I could truthfully answer, "no," to this question. It was surreal to buy long-term care insurance I would need if I became disabled one day and then immediately join my family to celebrate turning another year older. Before I went through the genetic testing process myself, my husband and I bought life insurance policies for each of our boys because they wouldn't be able to buy these policies later if I tested positive.

My younger brother's testing experience was vastly different than mine. Instead of meeting multiple times with a genetic counselor, he had one appointment with his general practitioner. His doctor ordered the bloodwork without any discussion about the pros or cons of getting tested, and my brother received his test result in an email. My younger brother tested negative, but I hate to think about anyone getting a positive result without the guidance and support a genetic counselor can provide. Testing positive is a life altering event – even if you've prepared for it – and it is crucial to have support in place to cope with the intense emotions that may follow. Carly was just one of the people I spoke with who felt they didn't have the support they needed during and immediately after this process.

Carly lives in Wales and has faced major challenges in recent years. She received her positive test result for Huntington's disease a few years after being diagnosed with another genetic disease that has left her almost completely blind. Her mom, aunt, and a cousin have since been diagnosed with the same eye disease. Carly and her cousin have lost their sight, but Carly's mom and aunt have not. Carly thinks having two genetic diseases makes her quite rare. "I'm intrigued to know if there's anyone in the world who's nearly blind and has tested positive for Huntington's," she said. "There aren't many people who fully understand all I have to deal with."

Before getting tested, Carly had a hunch she was going to get a positive result because she has a lot in common with her gene-positive dad. She wanted to know her gene status so she could participate in clinical trials if she tested positive. If she waited until symptoms arrived to learn her status, it would be too late to benefit from any potential treatment that participating in a clinical trial might offer. She also wanted to get tested early to give herself time to come to terms with knowing she is gene positive before symptoms appear.

Carly thinks going through the testing process during the COVID-19 pandemic made it especially hard to cope. COVID-19 restrictions did not allow meeting with a genetic counselor in person, so Carly felt like she had limited support throughout the process. Carly talked with a genetic counselor by phone several times over the course of many months to ensure she knew enough about Huntington's disease and was truly ready to get tested. She received her positive result during a brief phone conversation before being directed to the HD clinic for follow-up. The clinic's next available appointment was a month and a half away. In the meantime, Carly was on her own. There was no continuation of support from the genetic counselor after receiving her life-changing diagnosis. "I felt abandoned," she said.

In addition to going to the HD clinic, Carly sought support from a therapist, but it took her nine months to get an appointment. Until then, she coped on her own and considered giving up on pursuing her degree. "If you are considering genetic testing," she said, "get that support around you first. I thought I was prepared, but you're never prepared for what comes afterwards. It can take some time for it to sink in. If I could go back, I'd gather that mental health support before I got the result." Two years later, Carly's gene-positive result still consumes her. "It's been difficult to accept and come to terms with," she said. "Maybe I never will; maybe it will take a few years. Right now, I'm just dealing with it as positively as I can."

Carly doesn't regret knowing her gene status, but in hindsight, she thinks she tested for Huntington's disease at an inopportune time. She struggled to cope while also adjusting to losing her vision and while the COVID-19 pandemic was in full swing. "The mental health struggles after genetic testing are massive whether it's positive or negative," she said. "After the test result, it took a lot for me to persevere and find support, where I think it should just be an automatic thing. It's such a disappointment that you're kind of abandoned when you go through this massive life-changing thing."

Carly is grateful she can rely on her tightknit, supportive family, especially her mom who is one of her biggest sources of support. Carly was 13 years old when her dad tested positive. "For a few years, I blocked it out," she said. "But when my dad started getting symptoms, it was right there in front of me – something I saw daily." Since then, her dad has experienced cognitive decline and no longer drives. He's still able to walk, but he has constant chorea unless he's asleep. Now that Carly knows she's gene positive, she sometimes finds it hard to be around her dad because his symptoms cannot be ignored. "I completely adore my dad," she said. "I always have, but it can be quite tough for me to be around."

By the time Carly's dad tested positive, her aunt was already living in a nursing home. Carly and her dad both have a CAG repeat number of 42, but her aunt's repeat number was near 60. Carly's dad visited her aunt at the nursing home regularly despite the difficulty of seeing her decline – a preview of his own future decline. "It's quite remarkable," Carly said, "because even though my dad tested positive, he was there every week sitting by my aunt's bedside, watching TV with her, and feeding her. I can relate now because I've tested positive." Carly's aunt passed away in 2021 at the age of 59.

Carly has always considered herself a positive person, but that positivity has been hard to maintain in recent years. People often tell Carly she's a strong person, but that's not how she feels. "Nobody can be strong all the time," she said. "And if you're viewed as a strong person, nobody realizes that you are suffering. They disregard that. At the moment, I don't feel strong at all, even though I clearly am in some ways."

Knowing that she's gene positive, Carly is eager to do certain things sooner rather than later. Time moves quicker now, and she thinks a lot about what lies ahead. To avoid feeling overwhelmed, she does her best to focus on what's right in front of her, or she goes for a run or to the gym to ease negative thoughts. Working with her therapist helps her cope with anxiety. Carly finds it helpful to talk to someone outside her family because her mom is focused on caring for her dad, and her dad is coping with his own HD symptoms.

Being involved in the HD community also helps. As an HDYO ambassador, Carly works with her peers to raise awareness, educate others about Huntington's disease, and raise funds. She and her brother even did an assisted skydive to raise money. She's a member of HD-CAB, and she helps coordinate the HDYO Congress that takes place every two years. Participating in HDYO has been eye-opening and rewarding. "You don't realize how many people are going through the same thing until you get involved in something like this," she said. She's met people from all over the world and thinks they all benefit from connecting with each other. Carly now knows her experience in the United Kingdom is quite different from what people experience in other countries. While she has easy access to an HD clinic that provides ongoing support, some of her peers live in countries where Huntington's disease is poorly understood and where resources are scarce. She sees an even greater need in other parts of the world to increase awareness of Huntington's disease and garner support for those affected by it.

Carly has gained a lot of life experience in recent years. She has learned to be more patient, compassionate, and understanding. She is pursuing a master's degree in counseling and psychology, and she's doing well in school despite barriers related to being visually impaired.

While she doesn't know what her future holds, she knows she wants to do well at university, travel, and be happy. She'd also like to have children one day. She knows she needs to be patient. For now, she looks forward to finishing her degree so she can make a positive impact – something she is passionate about. "I've persevered, and I'm using my studies to help and support others," she said. "I don't want to see anyone else struggle the way I did." Helping others is the part of her future that gives her hope.

Despite the challenges of testing positive, Carly wants to ensure that something good comes out of her experience. "I would love to emphasize my hope and determination to not think of myself as having a death sentence and to not let my positive result define me," she said. "I want to focus on keeping my mental health – keeping my body and soul healthy. While I continue to have hope and determination, I will do all I can to fight back at this horrific disease despite my struggles."

Genetic testing aftermath

Knowing that my kids and I will not develop Huntington's disease removes an enormous burden from my life. My future is open-ended once again, and I have the rest of my lifetime to make plans and fulfill them. The same is true for my kids. I thought learning we did not inherit Huntington's disease would be one of the best days of my life, but immense relief was not my strongest reaction to my negative result. Instead, I felt an unexpected sense of loss. I had become a person at risk for Huntington's disease – it was a core part of my identity – so testing negative felt like giving up a piece of myself. It was surprisingly difficult, even though I was glad to see that part of myself go.

Once again, I had to define a new direction for my life. Now that I was no longer at risk for Huntington's disease, who was I? And why did I feel like I was abandoning my brother and his family, when that was far from the truth? It felt like we were no longer on the same journey. Despite a lifetime of HD experiences, testing negative makes me feel distanced from the HD community. I know I'm not an imposter, but I also know there are parts of the HD experience – testing positive, symptom onset, and disease progression – that will never be part of my own story.

After I tested negative, I was hesitant to tell my older brother. I worried about how he would feel when he learned that I get to live a life he will never have, and I worried about how my news would make him feel about his own situation. Even though gene status is determined at conception, and even though my brother had been having HD symptoms for years, I felt like this conversation marked a point at which my life took a sharp turn from his. There was no longer any doubt that we did not share the same future. We were on different paths, and I felt like my good news – my gain – highlighted his loss.

The aftermath of genetic testing is complicated no matter what the test reveals. Many people are surprised by how they feel once their result is known, especially if it doesn't match the result they expected. For those who test positive, the first year or two after testing, as well as the period when symptoms become noticeable, can be especially difficult. After learning their gene status, they may experience fear, depression, despair, anger, powerlessness, uncertainty, or numbness. They may feel a new sense of purpose, a greater appreciation of life, or a determination to maintain good health and accomplish life goals. They may feel all these things, and their feelings will likely change over time. Some people regret finding out their gene status, and many find they gain a deeper understanding of their HD parent. Despite the devastation of knowing they will develop Huntington's disease, people I spoke with emphasized that life is not over with a positive result or an HD diagnosis.

A research study that assessed how people feel after testing negative for Huntington's disease mirrored parts of my own experience. Many people have positive feelings – like relief and joy – that are countered by negative feelings – like disbelief and sadness. Many are uncomfortable being told they are lucky, and some feel pressure to live a good life to make up for those who cannot. Some people continue to search for HD symptoms in themselves even though they know they aren't there, and others question if their negative test result is accurate. This happened to my younger brother. He's not a worrier, and yet long after he tested negative, he thought he noticed HD symptoms and was compelled to check his paperwork to verify his negative result.

Some people who test negative regret choices they made when they were still at risk, like not investing in their future. This was the case for Samantha. It took her years to come to terms with her negative result. She grew up in New York, and her early childhood was a mix of instability and adventure. When Samantha and her sister were very young, their dad was an alcoholic, so their mom took the girls and left. For the next several years, they moved whenever Samantha's mom thought their dad might find them, which was often. "We were in and out of homeless shelters and welfare motels," Samantha said, "but my mom made everything fun. She would say, 'We're moving again! Start packing!' – like it was a fun thing to do. We probably moved 28 times. We could be living in a box, and we would make the best of the situation." Samantha knows they were often in unsafe situations, and she knows that her mom's family would have helped them in any way possible. Still, she values this period because of the time she got to spend with her mom.

Samantha's family never kept Huntington's disease a secret, but they didn't talk about it much either. "It was always like an elephant in the room," she said. "Everyone knew it was there, but no one spoke about it." Samantha always knew her grandpa and one uncle died of Huntington's disease, and her aunt died of Juvenile Huntington's disease. When Samantha was in sixth grade, her mom tested positive, and they moved in with family. "No one ever educated us about what it was. It just felt like, 'Okay, so mom's going to die.' When she got tested, that's all I knew." Samantha wanted to know more, so whenever she was assigned a school paper or project, she used that opportunity to educate herself about the disease.

Eight months after they moved in with family, Samantha's mom's physical symptoms progressed enough that she needed more care, so she moved to the Terence Cardinal Cooke Health Care Center in New York City. This center is one of a small number of long-term care centers in the United States that specializes in HD care. Samantha and her sister lived with an uncle for a few months before moving in with their dad who had been sober for many years by that time.

Samantha thinks watching her family members' decline is one of the hardest things about Huntington's disease. "I remember being upset because I couldn't hug my mom standing up," she said. "You start losing those little things that matter so much." When her mom could no longer talk, Samantha looked for other ways to connect with her. "You could always see what she was saying through her eyes," Samantha said. "She smiled through her eyes." Samantha is glad her mom always knew who she and her sister were.

Samantha's mom lived at Terence Cardinal Cooke until she died 12 years later, so Samantha became attached to many of the other residents and their families. She appreciates these relationships, but it's been hard to get to know and then lose so many people to the disease. One of her uncles also lived there for many years. Now that her mom is gone, mementos carry special meaning. Samantha's mom made several art projects at the hospital. On many of them, her mom wrote, "XOXO." Now, when Samantha and her sister exchange gifts, they often give each other items that say, "XOXO," in remembrance of their mom.

Despite her difficult experiences growing up, Samantha is in full support of others' decision to have kids if they're at risk or gene positive. "Why not?" she asked. "If that's what you want, I think people should support that." When Samantha was still at risk, however, she didn't want to have kids and have them go through what she did as a child of a gene-positive parent. Even so, Samantha said, "I wouldn't change a day with my mom. I'm glad I had the time I did with her."

Samantha receives a lot of support from her family. Samantha's sister, who is also her best friend, became a mother-figure to Samantha early on even though they're close in age. Their gene-negative uncle has also been a big source of support. He took in Samantha and her sister when their mom first moved to the hospital. He was a caregiver for many family members at one time or another and has watched multiple family members die from the disease. When this uncle tested negative, he told Samantha and her sister his news before sharing with the rest of the family, even his own kids. Samantha and her sister were still at risk, and he didn't want them to be caught off guard. He understood that his negative result might be hard for them to cope with.

Samantha didn't cope well with having Huntington's disease in her life. She and her sister attended one HD support group when they were young, but the room was full of older people so there was no one they could relate to. Samantha coped by turning to drugs and alcohol because that was something she could control. She also coped by shutting down emotionally, which she still tends to do. "I think having to deal with HD closed me off to showing my emotions," she said. After their mom died, Samantha and her sister attended an HDSA convention where Samantha learned about resources she wishes she had known about growing up. She started to feel knowledgeable about the disease.

After this convention, Samantha decided she was ready to get tested. She and her sister had agreed that if either of them decided to get tested, they would tell the other. When Samantha brought it up with her sister, however, she learned that her sister had already started the testing process. Fast forward several months, and the sisters were scheduled to get their test results two weeks apart from each other, with Samantha getting hers first. "The day before I was going to get my result, they called and said they would give us both our results together. Our whole family came," Samantha said, "but it was just me and my dad and my sister in the room." The three of them experienced a wide range of emotions while they waited. Knowing that both of his daughters were getting test results for Huntington's disease took a heavy toll on Samantha's dad, but he was there to support them as well as he could.

"They told us we were negative, and I was just stuck," Samantha said. "When we came out and told the rest of my family, everyone started crying." Samantha was happy her sister's result was negative, but she didn't know what to feel about her own negative result. Her initial reaction was, "What am I supposed to do with my life?" Before getting tested, she hadn't thought about what she wanted out of life if she was gene negative.

Samantha had only envisioned a life in which she would develop Huntington's disease. She lost all direction when that version of her future vanished, and she had difficulty coping with her negative result. "I had lived my entire life thinking I was going to have it," she said. "When I got the negative result, people were like, 'Oh my god, that's amazing!' It was the worst thing for me because I never finished college. I didn't take life seriously. Then I was like, 'I need to start putting lotion on my face!' You know what I mean? All the things I never thought of – like getting married or having kids – hadn't been in the cards for me."

When she was still at risk, Samantha used to be jealous of her gene-negative uncle and cousins. Since testing negative, though, she knows how hard it is to be on the other side. Sharing her news with her gene-positive cousins was tough. She sometimes wishes she could have the disease instead of them. "Obviously, it doesn't work that way," she said. "I'm going to cry just thinking about it… I can think about my life in a way they can't."

Adjusting to her gene-negative status took time. "If you think something for so long, it becomes a part of you, and a part of your life. My world got flipped upside down," Samantha said. "But in reality, I was digging myself a grave anyway." She was faced with either continuing the path she was on – where she coped by drinking alcohol and taking drugs – or making changes in her life to adjust to a future in which she would not develop Huntington's disease. It wasn't an easy choice. "It didn't change much about my life at first. It took me another two years to deal with it."

Samantha has been in a much better place since her family convinced her to go to rehab. "I started grieving and allowing myself to feel," she said. "Things are pretty great now." Samantha has been sober for five years, and she's now engaged. "Things are starting to happen in my life that I never thought could." Talking with others helps. Samantha knows she can go to therapy and talk to her AA sponsor, but when she wants to talk about her mom and Huntington's disease, she talks to family members or others in the HD community. Testing negative changed the way Samantha thinks about Huntington's disease, and it also changed the way she lives her life. "I had no hope when I was younger. Not an ounce of hope," she said. "Now, I do. I have a higher power in my life, so I definitely lean on Him a lot."

Samantha thinks there needs to be more HD advocacy, so she takes every opportunity to tell people about the disease. She periodically goes to Washington, DC, to advocate for changes in health policy, and she helps with an annual fundraiser for the care center where her mom and uncle used to live. When she shares her story, she's surprised by the number of people who approach her to say they have an HD connection. "We're a small community, but we're also big at the same time," she said. "Everyone wants to do whatever they can." Samantha is quick to say that she hates Huntington's disease, but she realizes her family would be different without it. "My family's story is how I became me," Samantha said. "We're all so close. I have the best family, you know. Not a lot of people can say that, and I'm grateful for that."

I am always aware that the life I get to live is nothing like the one I narrowly escaped but my brother did not – a difference caused by a small but distinct difference in our DNA. While dreaming about my future and its possibilities is a gift, it's hard to feel good about something my brother will never have. I think about how things would be different if our roles were reversed, or if he wasn't the only one of my siblings to be gene positive. My day-to-day life is different from my brother's and it's also different from that of his wife and kids. Their days are still dominated by Huntington's disease, so my life seems uncomplicated in comparison. I have conflicting feelings about being happy when I know they're all facing a difficult life, and I have guilt related to being *one of the lucky ones*,

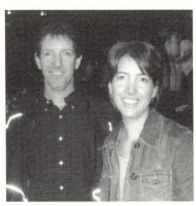

Me with my older brother – years before his HD diagnosis. Our lives look very different from each other now.

even though there is nothing about belonging to an HD family that feels lucky. I often feel like my gene-negative life needs to count for something. I owe it to others to do something constructive with the time I have.

I know these feelings are commonly known as *survivor's guilt*, but I wish there was another name for what I feel. For me, survivor's guilt implies that I'm at fault for something, but there is nothing I could have done to affect a different outcome. I cannot change my gene status, and neither can my brother. All I can do is live the rest of my life in a way that uses my experience and insight to move things forward. All I can do is put my *survivor's awareness* and understanding to good use and shine a light on the lived experiences of the HD community.

RESOURCES

About Genetic Testing

If you are thinking about getting tested for Huntington's disease or want to know more about the testing process, the HDSA website includes a *Genetic Testing Protocol for Huntington's Disease* document that describes best practices for HD genetic testing. The HDYO website has a *Genetic Testing Checklist* that suggests things to consider before, during, and after the testing process.

Getting Tested

To access genetic counseling and testing, it is recommended to work with a clinic with experience in genetic testing for Huntington's disease. An HD organization can help you identify these options. Members of the HD community in the United States also have an option to access genetic counseling and testing via telehealth through an organization called HD Genetics. This organization only serves the HD community, and it provides an anonymous testing option and financial assistance for those who need it.

In Vitro Fertilization with Pre-Implantation Genetic Diagnosis

HelpCureHD is a nonprofit that provides grants to help couples in the United States and Canada cover the costs of accessing IVF with PGD to prevent passing Huntington's disease to the next generation.

PROVIDING CARE

Growing up, I never imagined my family had a rare genetic disease, especially one like Huntington's disease. Not knowing we are an HD family meant my dad never got the help or compassion that could have made his life better. Not knowing meant my siblings and I all had kids before we learned we could pass on a genetic disease. Not knowing meant we didn't cherish the time we had with my brother before he started having HD symptoms. Unfortunately, ours is an all-too-common story. Many individuals and families with rare diseases face years of misdiagnoses and missed opportunities to receive appropriate care, something that has had a profound and lasting impact on my family and others.

I find myself wanting to blame my dad's doctors for not noticing my dad's chorea and not realizing my dad needed to see a neurologist. But Huntington's disease is just one of thousands of rare diseases – too many for medical professionals to be knowledgeable about all of them. Huntington's disease has a long list of potential physical, cognitive, and behavioral symptoms, many of which are common in other diseases. To complicate things further, not everyone with Huntington's disease has the same collection of symptoms. Early in the course of the disease, it is understandable that a physician might attribute a person's HD symptoms to another condition, especially when there is no known HD family history. Common misdiagnoses include, but are not limited to, Parkinson's disease, PTSD, schizophrenia, ADHD, or depression.

My brother has had good and bad experiences with medical providers and nonfamily caregivers, and his quality of life has been affected by how much those around him understand Huntington's disease. His second stay in a psychiatric ward is just one example. During this stay, he wasn't allowed visitors due to COVID-19 protocols, so he had almost no access to his family – the people who know him best and can advocate on his behalf. My brother's wife and kids were only able to wave at him a few times through a glass door. My brother was alone in an unfamiliar and frightening environment where there was little understanding of his disease. We had online access to his hospital chart, so we knew that staff often used restraints when administering his medication. I don't like to think about how scared he must have been.

While he was there, my brother's inability to use a cell phone further isolated him. When I called him on the hospital line, it was hard to know if he was still listening after being on the line for only a short amount of time. He answered one or two questions with short responses, but then it was quiet on his end other than hospital noises in the background. I don't know if he could hear me, but I talked for a while before hanging up. My brother withdrew deep within himself during this stay, and he seemed like a hollow shell when he was discharged more than two months later. It took him a long time to trust people again.

It is important to note that my brother's care also affects his family. This second stay in the psychiatric ward was emotionally challenging for his wife and kids. For me, too. Doctors made care decisions without consulting my sister-in-law, and she had to rely on daily hospital notes to understand how doctors and staff approached his care because there was almost no direct communication with her despite her efforts.

This experience was quite different from the care my brother receives in his current group home. It has a welcoming environment, and the owner communicates with my sister-in-law to brainstorm ways to accommodate my brother's needs. In this new setting, my brother and his family have settled into a new normal, and my brother is more at ease. He no longer seems lost and distant. He still experiences periods of decline, but changes in medication have been successful in addressing his symptoms. Our family's takeaway is that medical providers' knowledge of Huntington's disease and its symptoms, or their willingness to learn about the disease, has a direct impact on approaches to care, and thus the wellbeing of our loved ones.

Managing symptoms

Some HD patients are told that because Huntington's disease has no cure, they can't be helped, but a nothing-can-be-done attitude leads to missed opportunities to maximize an HD patient's quality of life. It is crucial for HD patients to have a team of professionals to manage symptoms and meet their wide variety of needs. Doctors can prescribe medications to address chorea and many of the disease's psychiatric symptoms. This comes with challenges, though. Some HD patients refuse medication because they don't like the side effects or because they don't notice their own symptoms. HD symptoms change as the disease progresses. Regular evaluation by a doctor with HD expertise is needed to ensure appropriate drugs and dosing are administered to maximize benefits and minimize side effects. Families should also be aware that some long-term care facilities overmedicate HD patients to make them easier to manage.

Physical, occupational, and speech therapists can help manage the many physical symptoms of Huntington's disease. These professionals can help patients adjust to changes in mobility, swallowing, and speech. They can also identify assistive devices, like specialty wheelchairs and beds, and suggest adaptations within the home to accommodate varied needs as symptoms progress.

Nonfamily caregivers and family members alike play a key role in managing an HD patient's daily care. People with Huntington's disease benefit when those around them are compassionate, respect them as a person, and try to keep them engaged in life. Some cognitive and behavioral symptoms can be better managed when there are established, simple, and predictable daily routines. If a person with Huntington's disease knows what to expect – when the world is easier to interpret and predict – there is less room for confusion and frustration. This approach can help minimize outbursts, too. A calm environment with minimal stimuli also helps.

When talking to someone with symptomatic Huntington's disease, it is important to remember it may take them longer to process information and respond. It can help to use simple requests, ask questions that only require yes-or-no answers, and allow an extended amount of time for a response. It is important for caregivers to remember that challenging behaviors are often caused by the disease itself and shouldn't be taken personally. When behaviors become challenging, it helps to remain calm and overlook small things. These approaches are simple, but they can help.

Many families, including my own, find that they have to educate medical professionals and nonfamily caregivers about Huntington's disease and advocate for better care and treatment for our loved ones. Jerry advocates on behalf of his wife, Terri, to ensure she receives the best care possible. Jerry, and their daughter, Abby, sometimes even request services or medication changes that are not automatically offered by Terri's doctors. Jerry and Terri live in Ohio, and Abby lives in California with her husband.

Terri was the first person in their family to be diagnosed with Huntington's disease. She was diagnosed in her mid-60s after having unexplained symptoms for many years. Neither of her parents had any indication of having the disease. She has late-onset Huntington's disease, which typically has a lower CAG repeat number and slower disease progression. It is also more likely to occur in individuals with no known family history. Abby tested negative soon after her mom's diagnosis. Abby's half-sister is at risk but is older than their mother was at symptom onset and suspects she may be gene negative. Huntington's disease may make a quick exit from their family.

Terri's first noticeable symptom was erratic driving. Jerry stopped riding with her about a decade before her diagnosis. "Whenever we went anywhere," he said, "I made sure I was driving because her foot was hitting the gas and letting up all the time. Awareness of her surroundings started to diminish. It was scary." After a yearlong conversation, and with help from other family members, Abby and Jerry convinced Terri to take a driving test. She eventually agreed and had to give up her driver's license and her independence. Terri's early symptoms may also have affected her work performance. She always performed well at work but rarely held a job for more than five years. She'd quit or get fired. When Terri was in her late 50s, she qualified for disability after developing neuropathy caused by chemotherapy. She hasn't worked since.

For Jerry, Terri's inability to manage money has been one of the more challenging aspects of Huntington's disease. As Terri's symptoms progressed, she began spending money freely and could no longer follow a budget. "She gets money and it's gone," Jerry said. "I know a lot of people spend to their limit, but with her, it was extreme." Jerry monitored Terri's spending closely and secretly put money into a 401(k) that Terri didn't know about to build up and protect their retirement savings. Now, he gives Terri a cash allowance every two weeks, and she has a credit card to charge small amounts. "That's the only thing that's kept us above water financially," he said. "The debt we've had to dig ourselves out of several times has been tough."

For Abby, her mom's behavioral symptoms have been especially difficult. Terri had outbursts for many years before her diagnosis, but she rarely had them around anyone other than Abby, Jerry, and Abby's half-sisters. Abby was very young when her mom's symptoms started. "I don't remember her as normal – without the outbursts or the irritability – and it slowly got worse," she said. Abby walked on eggshells around her mom, and she often wondered if her friends' moms screamed at them when no one was around. For a long time, Abby thought her mom had bipolar disorder. "Growing up, I didn't have a typical mom," she said. "Her cognitive decline and physical symptoms slowly progressed. It was hard to have a relationship, especially before I found out about HD."

Terri saw a psychiatrist for what they thought was ADHD, but she didn't get better. When Terri's changing symptoms could no longer be ignored, the family went in search of answers. It took almost five years to reach an HD diagnosis. "It was frustrating knowing something was going on but not knowing what it was or what to do about it," Jerry said. He turned to the internet for clues. "I started reading more and more, and thought, 'This Huntington's disease – everything they talk about fits almost to a T.'" Jerry advocated on Terri's behalf to get a referral to a neurologist. After a full neurological assessment, the doctor mentioned Huntington's disease, and Jerry knew immediately that his hunch had been right.

Proper medication has made a world of difference. Jerry thinks Terri is a lot more even-keeled now, but he sees less of her true personality as time goes by. "She was a go-getter," he said. "She could get things done. She hasn't had that capacity for a while. She still tries to organize things, but I have to circle back and make sure things like appointments are okay." Abby is glad she now understands the source of Terri's outbursts and other symptoms. "There was a lot of hurt from the way I grew up. I try to remember that she loves me," Abby said. "The good times remind me that she doesn't want to be that way or say hurtful things. She's such a positive, happy, giving, caring person. I can see she's not able to control her emotions. It's sad, but I feel like knowing she has Huntington's disease has been helpful." After Terri's diagnosis, Jerry and Abby both benefited from attending a support group where they could connect with others and talk openly about Huntington's disease.

Abby was 23 years old when her mom was diagnosed, and she knew right away she wanted to get tested. She was surprised to learn only a small percentage of people go through the predictive genetic testing process. "It blew my mind," she said. "I assumed because of the way I felt that it would be the opposite. I want to have kids one day, so I want to plan for that. I wanted to know." Abby's initial testing appointment was not what she expected. "I had an hour-and-a-half-long talk with the doctor. She tried to talk me out of it," Abby said. "I had done my research about getting tested, so I thought it was interesting that she didn't give both sides: this is why you might want to get tested; this is why you might not." Despite her doctor's discouragement, Abby went ahead with testing and received a negative result. "It was a relief, a lot of relief," Abby said. "I was scared, but in my heart, I knew it was going to be what it was going to be."

Terri is in her early 70s now. She can still walk independently, although slowly. She's no longer able to contribute to household chores, she sleeps a lot, and she has difficulty carrying out tasks from start to finish. Jerry retired early to keep a closer eye on Terri and take over more household tasks. Those changes have eased a lot of tension. Terri's ability to manage self-care is diminishing, though, and Jerry's efforts to encourage showering often trigger outbursts. "We may be getting close to the time when we need to ask for someone to come into the house to help her take care of things," he said, "because she doesn't want me to do that personal side of it."

Jerry feels fortunate that Terri's progression has been slower than what he sees in people with earlier disease onset, but he still doesn't like to think about the future. "As difficult as this is," he said, "I know how much worse it's going to get. There are times I hope it doesn't get too bad before the end comes. No one wants to see their loved one suffering, and thinking about the inevitable can be daunting. I've watched her slowly lose her independence, and I don't wish that on anyone. That's something I struggle with."

When describing his wife, Jerry said, "One thing about Terri is she's got the biggest heart of anybody. She's generous to a fault. People come to our house, and they can't leave without Terri giving them something. We've stuck together for 30 years, and we wouldn't have if there wasn't something good there. A lot of times, the negatives far outweigh the positives, but you just go on from day-to-day and month-to-month."

Terri has annual appointments at an HDSA Center of Excellence where she sees a neurologist and receives tips from physical, occupational, and speech therapists. At these appointments, Jerry finds it challenging to talk openly to the doctor or social worker. "I don't want to upset Terri when I say that these are things we need," he said. "I think she doesn't realize that she has shortcomings."

As a nurse, Abby feels comfortable asking for services she thinks will benefit her mom. HD patients are at high risk for falls, so Abby requested at-home occupational and physical therapy when her mom began having trouble maintaining her balance. Abby thinks her mom would also benefit from at-home visits from a speech therapist. "She's having more difficulty swallowing due to the progression of HD," Abby said. "She's been given a few strategies, but I still feel she would benefit from a speech therapist and more education. Choking and losing the strength to swallow increases the risk for pneumonia." Abby also advocated for her mom after a particularly bad outburst. She reached out to her mom's HD doctor who recommended a mood stabilizer. The medication also helps manage chorea. Instead of waiting to address concerns at annual appointments, Abby knows her efforts to advocate for her mom in between visits make a big difference in her mom's quality of life.

Even when things are challenging, Abby tries to maintain hope for her family's future. "Community gives me hope. Other people's stories give me hope. All the research that's being done gives me a lot of hope," she said. "When I think about how slow my mom's progression has been, it gives me hope that it will continue to be slow. I have to remain hopeful for my dad and also for my mom. We do the best we can."

Family caregivers

Providing care for a loved one with Huntington's disease is often a family affair. Family members become the first caregivers as a person with Huntington's disease gradually needs more assistance. There may be multiple family members from multiple generations needing care at the same time, and family caregivers themselves may be at risk, gene positive, or even symptomatic. Sometimes, a family member has to give up employment to devote time to their loved one's care, a change that can have a significant impact on family finances. These unique family dynamics add to the challenges of providing care for a loved one with a complex disease.

Caregiving duties can take a toll on mental and physical health. Family caregivers may feel overwhelmed and ill-equipped to take care of their loved one's many needs and manage any crises that arise. Caregivers must navigate challenging healthcare decisions such as whether to use a feeding tube and how to best approach end-of-life care. The stress of providing care can produce a wide range of emotions like anger, fear, anxiety, grief, and sadness. Caregivers may feel guilty if they move their loved one to a long-term care facility, even if they are no longer able to provide the level of care their loved one needs at home. Support from family, friends, and professionals is crucial, but many caregivers feel socially isolated and lack the help and resources they need. Family caregivers and loved ones with Huntington's disease can all benefit from seeing a counselor or therapist during challenging times.

In many HD families, children take on some responsibility for caring for their HD parent. They might be quite young when they start assisting with small tasks, and their caregiving duties may expand as they get older and as their HD parent's symptoms progress. The parent-child role eventually reverses as the parent needs more assistance and the child takes on more responsibility, a shift that can have an enormous impact on a child's life.

Children in HD families may find it difficult to balance home, work, and school responsibilities, and they may feel torn between providing care and living their own life. Caregiving responsibilities affect their decisions about whether to pursue postsecondary education, where to live when they are old enough to leave home, or even whether to go out with friends for an evening. Children may feel that caring for an HD parent takes priority over their own plans, even if family members tell them otherwise.

As they care for their HD parent, children know or eventually learn they may face the same disease one day. This experience is emotionally challenging, especially if their HD parent's symptoms are severe. As children enter adulthood, some distance themselves from this caregiving role, while others continue to actively participate in providing their HD parent with the type of care they hope to receive if they themselves develop Huntington's disease one day.

If a child is still performing caregiving duties when their HD parent passes away, the transition from being a caregiver to having free time to spend with friends can be especially challenging. I spoke with Amy just a few weeks after her mom died of cancer. She is an at-risk teen from England who was only seven years old when she started helping her family care for her gene-positive mom. She was struggling with how to transition to a life in which she was no longer a caregiver for the mother she loved dearly.

"My whole life has changed," Amy said. "All I've ever known is being a young carer." Amy talked at length about how hard it was when she felt like a parent to her mother and how alone that made her feel. Her friends didn't have the same kinds of responsibilities, nor did they worry about the future in the same way. Amy didn't have anyone to talk to who was also a young caregiver at risk for Huntington's disease. "Nothing scares me more than being at risk," she said, and then lightheartedly added, "I mean, I'm scared of spiders."

Amy captured the extensive effects of Huntington's disease succinctly. "It doesn't just affect the person," she said. "It affects the mind, body, soul. It affects their children, their future, their decisions in life, their dreams, their opinions – but it's such a slow process. You have to watch it happen right in front of you, and there's nothing you can do about it."

Before Amy's mom lost the ability to talk, she confided in Amy that she understood how hard it was for her. Amy recounted her mom's words during that conversation. Her mom said, "I want to look after you, but I know you're looking after me. I know how hard that is for you, and I didn't want that for you." Amy reassured her mom that having

Huntington's disease was not her fault, and she told her mom that she would continue to look after her. Even though Amy wasn't the only one caring for her mom, Amy's days were structured around caregiving duties. "My normal routine was get up, make sure mom's okay, go to school, pop home, look after mom," she said. Amy's weekends also centered around her mom's care.

Amy admires the way her dad cared for her mom. "I thank my dad for everything," she said. "He's the most patient person I've ever met. With everything that comes with HD – the screaming and shouting, all the troubled movements – it shows a lot about a person. I've never known anyone to love anyone the way my dad loves my mom. He stuck around for 22 years, even when he couldn't talk to her. He's always been here. A lot of people leave when their partner gets ill because they can't deal with it."

Amy's mom became ill with cancer and moved to a long-term care facility a few months before she died. Adjusting to life without her mom at home was difficult. While Amy's time was no longer structured around caregiving responsibilities, she still had constant thoughts about what her mom might need. "I'd worry about her when I was at school. Is she safe? How is she doing today? How's she feeling? I need to help her," Amy said. "I feel lost because my whole life was my mom. It's like a part of me has been taken away." Amy isn't sure how to fill her days. "I can do what I want now," she said. "I can go out with my friends and enjoy myself, but I don't know how to do it. I know it sounds stupid, but I don't know how to just be a teenager." When Amy does hang out with friends, she has a hard time enjoying herself. "I feel guilty sometimes for being happy. But even though I'm laughing and I'm happy, I'm not really happy." Her grief remains just below the surface.

Growing up in an HD family has influenced how Amy thinks about choosing a career. She first talked about wanting to be a counselor or social worker so she can help HD families and youth. Her family didn't receive a lot of support from her mom's doctors, so she'd like to fill that gap. Then, she talked about her dream of being a writer for a fashion magazine. When she talked about this potential future, her face lit up and her voice brightened, but she thinks choosing this option would feel like turning her back on the HD community.

Amy's dad encourages her to choose a career outside of the HD world. He'd like her to have at least part of her life that doesn't revolve around Huntington's disease. If she eventually learns she is gene negative, he thinks she could reconsider and switch to a career that uses her experience to help HD families. He also discourages her from getting tested and tells her, "Just live your life, Amy. Do what you want to do with your life." She knows this is because he cares about her.

Thinking about genetic testing is overwhelming for Amy. "The problem with HD," she said, "is you can get tested at 18, but you might not show any symptoms until 30, 40, 45. That means I'm going to have a cloud over my head for the next 10, 15, 20 years' time. I won't want the years to go by. It's scary." If she were to test positive, Amy thinks it would be hard to know there are things in life she won't be able to have – like a family. Amy sees the next 15 years as her only chance to live the life she wants, which is another reason she doesn't think she'll get tested right away. "Most people get 60 to 80 years now with modern medicine. I'm maybe getting 15 more years," she said.

For now, Amy thinks she'll wait to test until she's closer to the age her mom and grandma were at symptom onset, or she might get tested if she decides to have kids one day. "I think when I'm in my late 20s, 30, I will get tested. Because then I'll know that I've lived my life the way I've wanted to – that I've done things I want to do," she said. "I'm going to do what my dad's telling me: 'Just live your life.' If I have it, then I guess I'll just have to figure that out from there. If I don't have it, then that will be the best day of my life. Then I can have what I want in life."

Amy used to worry about what others would think if she told them her mom had Huntington's disease. "I was scared to tell people – not ashamed, because it's my mom. I was scared of what people would think of me or how they would treat my family or my mom," she said. "I always kept myself quite closed off from people, even my friends." Amy used to marvel at the normalcy she saw when she spent time with friends. "When I went to friends' houses, it was so weird to see normal parents doing normal things," she said. "My best friend's mom would ask me things like, 'What would you like for food, Amy? Do you want to do this or that?' – normal things that mothers ask and do. Even to see a mom just standing there normally and walking on her own – without any help, without wobbling, without movements, without struggling – has always been dead weird to me."

It has been hard for Amy to find people she can relate to. Her grandmother didn't develop HD symptoms until her kids were grown, so Amy doesn't have family members who understand what it's like to grow up with a symptomatic parent. Even her brother was a young adult by the time their mom was diagnosed. "A seven-year-old should be able to go to the park, spend time with their family, go to school, join their friends," she said. "I didn't have that life."

Amy joined a Facebook group for HD youth, but she still doesn't feel very connected to the HD community. She finds the most comfort in a video on the HDYO YouTube channel titled, *Huntington's Disease – The Impact on Young People*, that includes interviews with kids from HD families. "I relate to everything they say," she said. "To hear young people like me going through the same situation makes me feel less alone. Even though I've watched it about a million times, it makes me feel a little bit better."

Amy has a maturity that comes from being young when her mom was in the late stage of Huntington's disease. The experience has taught her a lot about herself. "If I didn't go through this experience, I wouldn't have become the person I am today. I wouldn't have become a stronger person," she said. "I wouldn't have been able to deal with situations in a better, mature, healthier way. I can always see the good in things because when the world has given you such darkness and hurt, you look for that light. I can understand people and what they're going through."

Amy shared the eulogy she gave at her mom's funeral. As she read, it was easy to sense how much she loved her mom and how much loss she has felt since her mom died. She summed up her mom's eulogy this way: "I talked about memories. I talked about my experience. I talked about the person she was, the impact she had on people, and how she inspired me to be strong. If my mom can be strong and brave and push through dealing with this awful disease, then I can deal with anything. If she can do it, I can do it. That's what I'm trying to do now."

A year and a half later, Amy was still grieving deeply for her mom. "I don't know how to move on in this new life," she said. Amy still feels guilty about trying to be happy, and even though her mom's HD symptoms were difficult to live with, she wishes she could go back to caring for her mom. But, for now, Amy continues to live life one day at a time. "I've learned that with grief, you have to push through every day and try to think of the good in the day to help you through. That's what I'm trying to do."

Transitioning to long-term care

My brother never moved back home after his first stay in a psychiatric ward. Instead, he moved to a group home, a move that was a huge adjustment for him and his family. My brother was no longer integrated into his family's home life, and nonfamily caregivers were now responsible for his daily care. Instead of interacting with each other throughout the day, my brother and his family had to settle into a new routine of family visits. I stay with my brother's family when I visit. After my brother moved to the group home, it was strange to be at his house knowing he no longer lived there. I half expected to see him when I walked in the door, even though I knew he was living somewhere else. The house felt like it was missing something – missing him. I had to visit many times before being there without him felt normal.

Some people with Huntington's disease remain at home for the duration of their disease, but many eventually need skilled nursing care. Transitioning to a long-term care setting is a significant change that is difficult for the person with Huntington's disease and family members alike. This transition is emotional and often takes place long after it becomes apparent that a higher level of care is needed or after family caregivers reach a point of exhaustion. It can also happen after a health crisis or psychiatric event. Sometimes, the physical layout of a house – a small bathroom or upstairs bedrooms – makes a family's home unsuitable for caring for a loved one in the later stage of the disease. Moving to a long-term care setting can be delayed, however, by wanting to keep a family member at home, a lack of access to quality care, or an inability to cover the cost of care.

Long-term care often involves a cycle of care in which loved ones move through a variety of settings. Options might include group homes, adult foster care, assisted living facilities, and skilled nursing facilities. This cycle of care may be punctuated by involuntary stays in psychiatric hospitals or state institutions if symptoms become severe and a person needs medication changes or round-the-clock monitoring. Changes in care may also be necessary if a current care setting can no longer meet a patient's needs.

There are many challenges related to accessing long-term care in the United States, including a limited number of long-term care facilities that specialize in providing HD care. In an online search, I found HD-specialized facilities in about a dozen states, not nearly enough to meet the needs of HD families. Adding to the challenge, few long-term care facilities are equipped to care for HD and JHD patients, and a standard nursing home is unlikely to have staff trained in caring for nonelderly residents or people with behavioral symptoms. Some facilities do not accept HD patients at all because of the high level of care required.

Other US facilities do not accept Medicaid, thus denying access for families who do not have private insurance or enough funds to pay out-of-pocket. Additionally, it can take several attempts for an individual to qualify for Social Security disability benefits, at which point there is an additional two-year waiting period before they can qualify for Medicare. In the meantime, families must find other ways to cover the high cost of care, something that can have a major impact on a family's financial situation.

Melissa has faced multiple challenges in identifying the best long-term care option for her husband, Dave, who was the first person in his family to be diagnosed with Huntington's disease. "At first, we were kind of on our own learning about this disease," Melissa said. In the last seven years, Dave has lived in several care settings, with each move being precipitated by an unexpected situation. "Maybe it's impossible," Melissa said, "but I wish I could have been a little bit prepared for the start of him needing outside care."

During the first few years after his diagnosis, Dave was unwilling to take medication to manage his symptoms. "When he started getting worse and became suicidal, that was when everything was suddenly put into motion," Melissa said. Two days after she reached out to an HD social worker about Dave's suicidal ideation, he was involuntarily committed to a psychiatric ward. When the ambulance came to their house, Dave went with the paramedics willingly. He even chatted with them. After he was admitted to the hospital, though, he didn't want to have any part of being there. His stay lasted one month.

Doctors overseeing Dave's care communicated little with Melissa. "I would work all day and go there at night and stay till 8 o'clock. I did that every day, but I didn't feel like I knew a lot about what was going on," she said. Doctors started Dave on medication and recommended an electrical brain stimulation procedure, something Dave refused. "Even though he was involuntarily committed," Melissa said, "they could not do that without his okay." After several failed attempts to convince Dave to agree to the procedure, the hospital told Melissa they could no longer help him.

Dave was still suicidal, so the hospital strongly recommended he not be left at home alone while Melissa was at work. Melissa had just a few days to find a long-term care option, something she hadn't anticipated. "I remember being totally overwhelmed when they said that. I hadn't thought ahead to when he left the hospital," she said. "Somehow, I thought they were going to make him better, he was going to come home, and everything was going to be fine."

With little time to make an important decision, Melissa hired a consultant to help her identify the best option. The consultant understood the complexities of accessing quality care and had an eye toward long-term financial planning. Paying for in-home care would have been expensive and would not have helped Dave qualify for Medicaid, something they were going to need in the long run. The consultant also determined that Dave and Melissa's home was not accessible for the wheelchair Dave had started using recently. Given his suicidal ideation, they were also concerned about the family's teenaged son who was still living at home. After taking these factors into consideration, the consultant recommended an adult family home as the next step.

The consultant and Melissa visited five adult family homes, some of which did not give Melissa a good feeling. She chose an adult family home whose owner had previously cared for a resident with Huntington's disease. She appreciated that the owner went to the hospital to meet Dave in person. The house seemed adequate, and the other residents were all men. It was the best fit. Over the next two years, Melissa used retirement savings to pay out-of-pocket for Dave's care. She worked with a lawyer to spend down their assets, pay off their house, and take other steps needed for Dave to qualify for Medicaid.

The transition to living in an adult family home was challenging because Dave didn't want to be there. "There was a rough transition period, obviously," Melissa said. "Every time I visited, he begged me to bring him home." Over time, Dave adjusted to his new home, and he and one of the other residents became friends. Melissa also had to adjust. "He was getting hard to live with, and it was getting stressful," she said. "He was drinking a lot, he had certain ways things had to be, and he was kind of rigid about things. It made me sad, but by that point, things were so bad between us that it was honestly a relief. I no longer had to worry about doing something that was going to upset him. It felt strange at first, especially when he was in the hospital. Everything was surreal. I remember feeling so guilty about what I had done. I still do."

Melissa often has to explain Huntington's disease to Dave's doctors and nonfamily caregivers. While the owner of the adult family home had previous experience caring for an HD patient, Melissa thinks that patient was in the late stage of the disease. Now that she knows more about Huntington's disease, she realizes that working with a patient who is bedridden is different from working with a person like Dave, who is in the middle stage of the disease and has challenging behavioral and cognitive symptoms. "They hadn't seen all this other stuff," she said. "Even when somebody says they've got experience, that doesn't mean they know what it's going to be like. Even I didn't know what changes were coming. Asking more questions about what they had done to care for that previous person would have been a good idea. I naively thought, 'Oh, he's taken care of someone. Awesome. This is great.'"

Unfortunately, caregivers at the adult family home had trouble getting Dave to comply with their requests. "They didn't know how to deal with the hard stuff," Melissa said. "He went so long without showering, and they didn't know how to work with him to take medications. They always defaulted to asking me to try to get him to do those things, which I was happy to do, although I wasn't always successful. Now, though, I realize that's not my job." She also realized that the caregivers' reliance on her to solve problems let them off the hook – they weren't motivated to learn about Huntington's disease or take responsibility for addressing Dave's changing needs. As Dave's needs increased, Melissa felt less and less like his spouse. "I've crossed over to where I feel more like a caregiver. It would have been nice not to have to play that role."

When Dave began refusing medication again, a nurse practitioner for the adult family home alerted Melissa that Dave's condition was worsening. The nurse practitioner told Melissa he might need a change in care, possibly a nursing home. Melissa reached out to several nursing homes and was told that Dave's condition did not warrant full-time nursing care. Melissa was surprised that the nurse practitioner and the house doctors all recommended this type of move when it didn't match Dave's needs. Still, she continued to look for an alternative care setting.

Just months later, Melissa received a call from the owner of the adult family home who told her Dave had tried to run his wheelchair into another resident. He was now considered a danger to others. Melissa wonders if Dave's chorea was to blame, especially because he refused to take medication that could lessen his movements. The owner told Melissa he was calling 911. At the emergency room, doctors assessed Dave and saw no need to admit him. "The house wasn't going to take him back," Melissa said. "So, I was supposed to take him home? I felt blindsided. He didn't need to be admitted, but he needed a better place to go." Melissa knew their home was not set up to accommodate Dave's needs. She felt stuck.

Dave was eventually admitted to the hospital's psychiatric ward because there was no other option available to him. Months later, Melissa was asked to meet with Dave's care team. Again, Melissa was told she had a few days to find Dave a place to live. The hospital had done all they could for him, and the hospital social worker gave Melissa a short list of potential adult family homes. All of them were at least an hour's drive away from home and none seemed like a good fit. The social worker was unwilling to look further, so Melissa was on her own.

Melissa quickly identified adult family homes closer to home and visited several in person. When she met with the owner of Dave's current adult family home, it was clear that it was a suitable place, and the owner was open to meeting Dave's needs. "She was the only one who was concerned about making sure he was in the right situation for him and that it was going to work out for the caregivers – for everybody," Melissa said. "She made sure this was going to be a good fit. You would think that would be obvious, but no."

The adult family home also had a mental health certification, so the owner made sure she could line up extra mental health services for Dave before she would accept him. Owners from the other adult family homes on Melissa's list didn't ask many questions about Dave and became irritated when Melissa didn't immediately say she would take an open spot. They seemed more concerned with filling a vacancy than making sure they could provide the right kind of care.

While caregivers at the first adult family home relied on Melissa to aid in Dave's daily care, she's had a completely different experience at Dave's new home. "They default the other way," she said. Melissa can only recall one instance in which they called and asked for her assistance when Dave refused a blood draw. She assured the owner that she is willing to help anytime but was told the caregivers need to know how to care for Dave when Melissa is unavailable. "They told me it's their job, and they need to figure out what works," she said.

All residential care options have pros and cons, but Melissa is mostly happy with Dave's current adult family home. "I like the caregivers who chat with him," she said. "You can tell the ones who are more comfortable with him. I like it when they involve him or try to find out what his past life was like. Sometimes I'll say something about him, and they'll be like, 'Oh really?' Then they'll ask questions. I want them to recognize that he used to be just like everyone else. He used to do all kinds of things."

Melissa copes with Dave's Huntington's disease, including decisions related to his care, by compartmentalizing her thoughts. "I do try to put this kind of thing out of my mind because I have to cope," she said. "I spend so much time trying to feel like life is normal: 'We're gonna go visit your dad. We're gonna have dinner. This is normal life.' When I start thinking about the future, I get too overwhelmed. When I think about the past, I get too sad realizing how much he's lost and how much our lives have changed. I just have to think about the present. What can he do right now? What makes him happy? Trying to plan for the next crisis doesn't work well mentally."

Melissa knows her previous experience may not help if she needs to find another new place for Dave. "If I had to find another house for him, it wouldn't necessarily be any easier than the first two times," she said. "There's still a learning curve. It would still be super stressful, and I wouldn't feel like I knew what I was doing. Maybe you can't prepare for this kind of thing. You don't see it coming." Melissa's goal is to keep Dave happy and comfortable. Again, focusing on the present helps. She does what she can to make Dave's life as good as possible. When she recently brought Dave a milkshake, his face lit up. "Even before he tasted it, he had this cute little smile. They are awesome milkshakes. This disease makes you appreciate those little things a lot more."

Quality care

The physical, cognitive, and behavioral symptoms of Huntington's disease can be difficult for caregivers to work with, especially if they know little about the disease. When I was still at risk, it was frightening to think about what it would be like to have a disease that others didn't understand and to be cared for by people who were not trained to manage its symptoms. What would it be like to have difficulty interpreting the world around me and not be able to clearly communicate with the people responsible for my care?

While the knowledge needed to care for an HD patient over the course of their disease could fill volumes, any amount of effort to understand the person and their disease can go a long way toward improving an HD patient's quality of life. People with Huntington's disease may become fearful, combative, or anxious when care approaches don't accommodate their unique needs; and they may be more relaxed and easier to care for when the care environment takes their needs into account. Carina Hvalstedt is a psychiatric nurse who understands the importance of tailoring care to a patient's needs. She serves on the board of the Swedish HD organization, Riksförbundet Huntingtons Sjukdom, and she has worked with the HD community for two decades. She focuses on supporting all family members, but especially children.

Interacting with many people in the HD community has broadened Carina's understanding of Huntington's disease. She has learned that what is true of one person with the disease isn't necessarily true of another. Even after decades of experience, she continues to learn new things. If someone tells Carina they understand Huntington's disease because they've met one or two people with the disease, she knows they still have a lot to learn. Carina emphasized that it's important not to confuse a person with their disease. "They are not HD," she said. "They are a person who has HD. Each person has different symptoms."

Carina opened her own private care home in March 2022 after recognizing the need for specialized care for people with Huntington's and related diseases. Her care home has 12 apartments plus common areas where residents have meals and activities, and it is equipped to provide daily and end-of-life care. It has wide corridors to allow plenty of room for those with Huntington's disease to find their balance within a larger space. For some people with chorea, this can be a better way of maintaining balance than using a walker.

Carina's care home incorporates elements she thinks are important to maximizing residents' quality of life. "You need to make it like a home, not like a care home," she said. She described colors and artwork and floor-to-ceiling windows with views of nature. "It's calm, and people become calm when they come here," she said. Residents benefit from being with others with the same disease. No one stands out as being different. "Everybody understands, even if they have different symptoms."

Many people with Huntington's disease have irregular sleep patterns, but most residents at Carina's care home sleep well. She attributes this to adjusting routines to suit residents' patterns. Not everyone gets up or eats breakfast at the same time. "They can sleep as long as they want to," she said. "We have breakfast at 10 o'clock. Some of them have perhaps had one or two breakfasts because some of them are awake at 5 o'clock. If they are hungry, they are hungry. A lot of care homes are strict about mealtimes. You need to have another way of looking at people. They are in their homes." This approach – along with comfortable beds, sleep medication if prescribed, and eating before bedtime to avoid hunger during the night – has resulted in most residents sleeping from 9 or 10 o'clock at night to 8 o'clock in the morning. One resident is often awake for long periods during the night, but that's the exception rather than the norm.

Carina is in tune with the unique needs and symptoms of HD patients. She noted that people's eyes are affected early in the course of the disease. Eye muscles become less flexible, resulting in jerky movements that are hard to control. Eventually, this makes it hard for someone with Huntington's disease to see what's happening in their peripheral vision. "This is a small thing, but it's a big thing," Carina said. If a caregiver moves toward an HD resident from the side with a bite of food, for example, the resident might be surprised when the food enters their field of vision. A natural HD reaction might be an exaggerated chorea movement of the arms, which can be misinterpreted as an indication that the person doesn't want the food. A better approach when feeding a person with Huntington's disease, or providing personal care like brushing teeth, is to be directly in front of them and explain what's happening as it happens. No surprises.

People with Huntington's disease can be easily distracted and sensitive to loud noises. Distraction can make eating difficult, especially for people who already have difficulty swallowing and are prone to choking. Noise and stress should be minimized, and some people benefit from eating in a separate room or at a different time. "When you are feeding someone, find a way to do it with respect," Carina said. "And try to give them things they like to eat. That's important."

HD patients are also sensitive to physical sensations. Bathrooms can be echoey with loud toilets and running water, and shower spray can feel harsh on the skin, so it makes sense that some people with Huntington's disease don't like to shower. Strategies to accommodate these sensitivities include placing a sock over the showerhead to soften the spray and washing the feet first so the person can feel the water before moving on to other parts of the body. Allowing a person to do as much of their own self-care as possible and talking through the steps is helpful. Again, no surprises. Carina suggests that caregivers talk to an HD patient about setting out clothes in the evening to be ready for a shower the next day, and then place a sign on the bathroom door that says, "Shower," as a reminder. The goal is to create a predictable and low-stimulation environment.

"It's important to have carers specialized in Huntington's disease," Carina said. "That's also important for relatives, so they don't have to explain everything." She encourages caregivers to think about how an HD patient's cognitive and behavioral symptoms affect how they interpret their world. For example, people with Huntington's disease often need more time to process a request before they can provide an answer or switch to a new task. When things change too quickly, HD patients may experience stress or anxiety that can aggravate chorea. Carina tries to find ways to avoid that.

Central to Carina's approach is creating an environment where a person with Huntington's disease feels seen. "It's important to know their opinion," she said. "They mean something to you. See the person – that's my advice. I'm keen on caring, so I think it's important to see how you can provide care and how you can find the person in the care. Try to make their life as good as you can." Carina emphasized the importance of considering the person behind the disease. "You need to be curious to see who they are behind the mask," she said. "How can I get in contact?"

Carina encourages caregivers to think through what they would do if they were at risk for Huntington's disease so they can better understand their patients. "Should I do the test? Should I not do the test? How would I react, and how would it be for my family, for my siblings, and so on? When you're working with people with Huntington's disease," she said. "I think you should have asked yourself those questions to understand the difficulties a family is living under, and the worries." Carina cautions caregivers against trying to diagnose a patient's relatives. "It's a lot of speculation," she said. "Have they tested? It's important to keep that to yourself. It's not good for the person in your care if you say, 'I see that your daughter has symptoms.'"

In addition to opening her own care home, Carina has worked with a team to develop a one-hour online basic training module for caregivers called, *Basic Training on Huntington's Disease*. It is available in English and Swedish on the Riksförbundet Huntingtons Sjukdom website. With support from the European Huntington Association (EHA) and the European Huntington's Disease Network (EHDN), the team is securing funding to translate a more in-depth course into English and additional languages.

The basic training module provides an informative explanation of HD symptoms that would be useful for anyone working with HD patients. It provides strategies to address temper outbursts, ease communication difficulties, and help patients perform daily tasks. Suggested strategies include reducing stimuli, establishing simple routines, learning about the disease and how it affects all members of the family, proper use of medications, and treating people as if they matter. The training encourages caregivers to start from a place of understanding and anticipating needs rather than responding to symptoms as they arise.

If I had inherited Huntington's disease, I would likely be in the middle stage of the disease now, or maybe even the late stage. It's possible I would live in a long-term care setting where I would be much younger than other residents. I would rely on others to help me shower, get dressed, use the toilet, eat, and turn on the television. I may or may not be able to effectively communicate with those around me, and I would only see my family when they came for a visit. I wouldn't leave my residence on my own. I can only hope that I would have caregivers who are kind, patient, willing to learn about my disease, and content to perform a tough job. In addition, I would hope that my caregivers are treated well, sufficiently compensated, and not overworked – important factors in retaining high-quality caregivers. This scenario is hypothetical for me, but these are the foundational pieces of my brother's day-to-day care needs.

HD patients need care for a long time, and providing care for someone with physical, cognitive, and behavioral changes is challenging. Accessing appropriate care for our loved ones is essential to maximizing their quality of life, but it is not easy to find affordable, high-quality long-term care settings that are set up to meet their needs. One of the *Livable Lives* storytellers dreams of creating a residential community where HD patients can live communally and receive support and specialized care. Perhaps it would be a village of tiny homes where HD patients could move about freely and have a sense of normalcy within a safe environment. I like to imagine this setting where Huntington's disease is accepted and not out of the ordinary.

It is clear to me that providing quality care for our HD loved ones requires much more than managing symptoms. It also includes treating patients with dignity, maximizing patients' quality of life, supporting family caregivers, and ensuring medical professionals and nonfamily caregivers are familiar with the disease. Above all, it is important for medical professionals and nonfamily caregivers to know that our loved ones are people to know and respect, not a problem to solve or keep quiet. Our loved ones deserve care that allows them to make the most of their livable lives.

RESOURCES

To understand and access available care options, consult with a physician, a healthcare social worker, and/or an HD organization. The following is a small selection of what's available to help families and caregivers provide care for someone with Huntington's disease.

Care Strategies and Approaches

Many HD organization websites provide caregiver guides with information that is useful for family members, family caregivers, and nonfamily caregivers alike. Many HD organizations also have social workers on staff who can provide education to caregivers.

The Swedish HD organization, Riksförbundet Huntingtons Sjukdom, has a one-hour online training module for caregivers called, *Basic Training on Huntington's Disease*. It provides an easy-to-understand overview of the disease along with approaches to caring for HD patients. It is available on the organization's website in Swedish and English and will be translated into other languages.

HD educator and advocate, Jimmy Pollard, wrote a book called, *Hurry Up and Wait! A Cognitive Care Companion: Huntington's Disease in the Middle and More Advanced Years*, that outlines strategies for communicating with and caring for someone with Huntington's disease. The book includes a set of exercises to help readers understand the cognitive impairments caused by the disease.

OTHER CARE TOPICS

Consult with your local or national HD organization for country-specific resources for long-term care options and guidance for qualifying for disability benefits, need-based financial assistance, and other help.

The Conversation Project website provides access to a workbook titled, *What Matters to Me*, that helps people with serious illnesses identify their priorities for health care and quality of life.

HDSA, Help4HD, and other HD organizations provide HD-specific resources for law enforcement, social workers, genetic counselors, occupational and physical therapists, and other service professionals to help them better serve the HD community.

RESEARCH

Members of the HD community often express hope that researchers will find a treatment or cure before a family member, or they themselves, develop symptoms or experience disease progression. As we wait for treatments to be developed, however, loved ones continue to become symptomatic, decline, and pass away. Even with medications to ease chorea and some of the disease's behavioral symptoms, Huntington's disease can be difficult to manage. Scientists pinpointed the genetic mutation that causes Huntington's disease more than 30 years ago, but families are still waiting for something – anything – that will slow or halt disease onset and progression and extend the amount of quality time we have with our loved ones.

The HD community is not alone in looking to research as a source of hope. Huntington's disease is just one of more than 6,000 rare diseases that affect more than 300 million people worldwide. Almost three-quarters of these diseases are genetic, and only one-tenth have an FDA-approved treatment. There are large gaps to be filled to address the research and treatment needs of the HD and rare disease communities.

Still, there are reasons to be hopeful about HD research. There is a large and growing number of research studies in progress, and HD researchers have systems in place to recruit participants for their studies.

In addition, pharmaceutical companies have taken an interest in understanding Huntington's disease from the patient's point of view, an important development that will improve patient outcomes when treatments become available. Despite these developments, movement forward is slow. Research takes a lot of time, something those in the HD community do not have.

Laboratory research

While scientists know the exact location of the genetic mutation that causes Huntington's disease, finding a treatment or cure is far from straightforward. There is a lot to unravel and understand. Long before researchers conduct clinical trials with human patients, the process begins with understanding the basic science of Huntington's disease and identifying potential treatments through preclinical research in a laboratory setting. In the lab, researchers are seeking better ways to define and detect disease onset because changes can be seen in brain scans years before measurable HD symptoms appear. Researchers are expanding our knowledge of how the disease affects parts of the body outside the brain, and how the disease progresses, including how other genes may impact that progression. They are also looking for ways to prevent or significantly slow nerve cell death and deliver potential drugs or treatments to the brain. These are just some of the many avenues of research taking place.

To learn more, I spoke with three researchers from the College of Medicine and the Psychology Department at Central Michigan University (CMU). Dr. Gary Dunbar and Dr. Julien Rossignol co-direct the Field Neurosciences Institute Laboratory for Restorative Neurology, which is part of the Brain Research and Integrative Neuroscience (BRAIN) Center. Dr. Bhairavi Srinageshwar is a postdoctoral researcher in their lab. Their HD research focuses on delivering gene editing tools to the brain, increasing neuroprotective molecules in the brain, and using stem cell therapies.

The goal of preclinical research is to prove concepts in a controlled environment before moving on to clinical trials that include human subjects. It can take two or three years for preclinical studies to generate results, and researchers must proceed through many steps to determine if research in the lab might also help humans. "We need to test so many variables," said Dr. Rossignol. "What works on cells, rats, and mice, might not work on humans."

Obtaining funding and conducting research both take a considerable amount of time, and the journey from an idea to the laboratory to a clinical trial can be halted anywhere along the way. However, each step provides new information and refines the research focus, especially if corrections need to be made. "It doesn't happen overnight," said Dr. Srinageshwar. "It happens in stages. The good thing is that we can learn what went wrong. From that, we can design a better experiment. It's a learning experience."

CMU researchers are studying CRISPR-Cas9, a gene editing tool that may one day be used to snip out the extra CAG repeats that cause Huntington's disease. If successful, it would directly target and correct the genetic mutation at its source. CRISPR-Cas9 has revolutionized the field of gene therapy. "There's a lot of hope in that line of research," said Dr. Dunbar. "Some of the initial gene therapy trials in humans did not work out so well, but I think it's only the beginning of what can be done. As we get better at it – particularly using animal models – it will ultimately materialize into an effective treatment."

Scientists may one day learn to correct the mutation that causes Huntington's disease in one cell in a laboratory setting, but correcting the mutation in billions of cells in a human body is a different matter, and correcting the mutation in dying brain cells may be even more challenging. Once scientists learn how to successfully deliver gene editing technology to the brain and remove or replace the extra CAG repeats in brain cells, they will need to conduct additional studies to determine if doing so causes any detrimental effects. These are just some of the challenges scientists need to address before this technology can benefit the HD community.

CMU researchers are also looking for ways to increase the amount of GM1 ganglioside in the brain. GM1 ganglioside is a fatty sugar molecule that plays a role in protecting neurons from damage. People with Huntington's disease have lower amounts of GM1 ganglioside in their nerve cell membranes, which may contribute to some of the cognitive decline associated with Huntington's disease. Finding a way to restore GM1 ganglioside to a normal level could help protect cognitive ability. "GM1 ganglioside has been used in clinical trials with Parkinson's patients with some success," said Dr. Dunbar. "We're thinking this could be fast-tracked. We could probably have this in the hands of Huntington's patients long before the gene therapy would be ready, so we've been working hard on that one." Interestingly, the GM1 ganglioside used in the CMU lab comes from sheep raised by a nonprofit called Shepherd's Gift, which was started by a group of families with friends and relatives with Huntington's disease.

Another line of research at CMU is examining stem cell therapy as a means to slow HD progression. CMU researchers developed a strategy to transplant a type of stem cells that can reduce inflammation and protect neurons. These stem cells can be genetically altered to produce more of a molecule called brain-derived neurotrophic factor (BDNF) that could slow neurodegeneration caused by Huntington's disease.

While CMU researchers are expanding our knowledge of Huntington's disease through laboratory research, their efforts to create a research culture that teaches young scientists to care about the people who will one day benefit from their work is just as influential. Soon after arriving at CMU, Dr. Dunbar met a couple who were involved in the HD community. They helped him see the importance of getting to know people with the disease. Dr. Dunbar got involved and even served as a scientific advisor for the Michigan chapter of HDSA for many years.

"When they connected me with Huntington's patients and families in Michigan, I was hooked," Dr. Dunbar said. "I was adopted as part of the Huntington's family right away. I've lost a lot of friends to Huntington's now, a lot of friends. You want to do everything you can to stamp out this devastating disease because people's lives depend on it." Dr. Dunbar has great admiration for the many family caregivers he's met. "When I see those who have stuck it out with their spouse and their kids," he said, "the triumph of the human spirit is unlike anything I've seen."

Many researchers never meet people with the diseases they study because they focus on the science of the disease. When Dr. Rossignol was doing his PhD research, he studied Huntington's disease as a vehicle to advance the field of stem cell research. It wasn't until he was invited to a large HD event that he began to see how much his research could impact HD patients and families. At that event, Dr. Rossignol was asked to answer questions about his research in layman's terms. As he spoke with people affected by Huntington's disease, he was asked repeatedly when there was going to be a treatment or cure. He realized his research could have a much bigger impact than just learning about stem cells.

These connections to the HD community motivate Dr. Rossignol when his work is challenging or frustrating. "It makes me want to work more," he said. "I understand what the patients and families are waiting for and why it's important to come to the lab. That's why we do what we do. When you start as a graduate student, you want to work in the lab – it's fun, but what does it mean? I always tell my students that the families and patients expect a lot from you." To give their students the same kind of connection to the HD community, Drs. Dunbar and Rossignol take them to the annual HDSA Team Hope Walk. Dr. Rossignol encourages students to talk to and connect with HD patients and families and tell them about their research. These interactions help students see how their research and studies relate to real people.

Dr. Rossignol also asks his students to consider what they would do if they had to decide whether to get tested for Huntington's disease. Usually, about 40 percent of students say they would go ahead with predictive genetic testing. Then, Dr. Rossignol spends time helping students think through why only a small percentage of people at risk for Huntington's disease seek out predictive genetic testing. Connecting students with the HD community and asking them to consider what it would be like to have Huntington's disease in their own lives is important. Some of these students are studying medicine and may work with patients someday, so having a better understanding of the HD community will make them more effective researchers and clinicians.

Dr. Srinageshwar is a good example of a researcher who has stepped outside of the lab to have an impact on HD families. In addition to attending fundraising walks with her colleagues and students, she also volunteers for HD organizations. She serves as an HDYO ambassador, and she is a mentor with the Youth and Young Adult Mentorship Program, which is a partnership between HDYO and HDSA. As a member of HDYO's education and research committee, Dr. Srinageshwar also helps produce videos and website content to communicate new research findings to a general audience. Through these efforts, Dr. Srinageshwar has made connections within the HD community that have taught her about the personal impacts of Huntington's disease – something she would not have gained from lab work alone. "It has truly been an eye opener," she said.

Each of these researchers gains inspiration from families and individuals impacted by Huntington's disease. When asked what he would like to convey to the HD community, Dr. Dunbar replied, "I always try to instill hope. There are thousands of researchers out there trying to find effective treatments and a cure, and every day we learn something new. Every day – even if it's just an inch closer – we're getting there. It's going to happen. I'm convinced of that."

Research that includes HD patients

Participating in research of any kind empowers those in the HD community by allowing them to be part of the search for a treatment or cure. The HD community can take part in two kinds of research: observational studies or clinical trials. Observational studies track information gathered from surveys, neurological assessments, cognitive tests, blood samples, spinal taps, and other measures to learn more about Huntington's disease. This information helps researchers understand changes that occur in the brain and body before and after symptom onset.

Enroll-HD is the largest observational study with more than 20,000 participants from five continents. Participants can be gene positive, gene negative, at risk, or HD family members. Participants visit an Enroll-HD site in-person once a year to complete a battery of assessments that measure motor function, behavioral and cognitive function, ability to complete daily tasks, and quality of life. Information gathered through Enroll-HD provides a big-picture overview of Huntington's disease that can identify gaps in support, explore measures of disease progression, and inform clinical trial design. Enroll-HD also serves as a patient registry system from which researchers can recruit participants for research studies.

Once a potential drug or therapy shows promise and is proven safe in a laboratory setting, it can then move on to clinical trials with humans. Clinical trials have three distinct phases: phase 1 tests a potential treatment in 20 to 100 people to assess safety and dosage; phase 2 examines effectiveness and side effects in up to several hundred people; and phase 3 further examines effectiveness and monitors for adverse reactions in 300 to 3,000 people.

There are many HD clinical trials currently underway to test drugs that have the potential to better treat chorea, lower or inhibit production of the toxic huntingtin protein, prevent neurodegeneration, improve or protect cognitive function, and address behavioral symptoms. One challenge for HD clinical trials is the slow progression of the disease. To evaluate the effects of a potential drug or therapy, researchers must track changes over a long period of time, thus slowing the pace of research.

Most drugs tested for brain diseases never make it all the way through the clinical trial process. Clinical trials can be halted at any point if there are safety concerns or if a treatment does not appear to provide any benefit. The HD community's hope in research was shaken in 2021 and

2022 when several closely watched HD clinical trials were halted. One was a gene therapy study, and the others focused on lowering levels of the mutant huntingtin protein in the brain. Reasons for halting these studies included adverse side effects, not achieving anticipated outcomes, or having an unfavorable risk-benefit profile. These clinical trials were highly anticipated by the HD community, and many people thought there would be a breakthrough in finding a treatment or cure. When that hope was crushed, many found it difficult to cope. Several HD organizations launched outreach campaigns to support the HD community and help them be better prepared for the ups and downs of clinical research.

While disappointing, a halted research study is far from a failure. Researchers learn from every step of the process, even when findings are inconclusive or produce unanticipated results. Knowing what doesn't work is just as important as knowing what does. Depending on initial results, some halted studies can be redesigned and go through the clinical trial process once again. One of the recently halted studies found that patients who were younger and less symptomatic may have benefited from the study drug. So, a year after halting the original clinical trial, researchers were back on track with a new clinical trial for this targeted population.

The research landscape continues to change and move forward, and several clinical trials announced encouraging results in the summer of 2024. Due to the amount of time it takes to conduct research and the setbacks that can occur, a high volume of research is essential for eventual success in treating Huntington's disease. It's unlikely that a single drug or treatment will be all that is needed to treat Huntington's disease. Even for a more common neurodegenerative disease like Alzheimer's disease, researchers are a long way from identifying an easy-to-take pill that halts disease progression. There are now FDA-approved drugs for Alzheimer's, but they do not cure Alzheimer's, and they can be expensive and invasive.

Every day counts for members of the HD community, and a treatment or cure cannot come too soon. Rob Haselberg knows this all too well. He works for a gene therapy company that focuses on neurodegenerative diseases like Huntington's disease and ALS. Rob has many roles within the HD community. He serves on the boards of the European Huntington Association and Vereniging van Huntington (the Dutch HD association). He is a patient representative on the steering committee for clinical trials for a drug called tominersen, and he is a member of HD-CAB. Rob also speaks publicly about Huntington's disease to raise awareness.

Rob, his brother, and several of his cousins are gene positive. Rob's family members tend to have late-onset Huntington's disease. His grandma lived to 80 years old, and his mom, who is in her early 70s, is in the late stage of the disease. Rob had already moved away from home when his mom started having symptoms, but his younger brother had not. Their mom has never been an easy person to be around. "She has a personality," Rob said, "and she's not afraid to show it, let's say. I've never been on the receiving end, but my brother has. If she had tantrums or anything, she took it out on him, especially early in her disease. She had moods like bipolar, and she was verbally aggressive, physically aggressive."

Rob was working on his PhD in chemistry when his mom tested positive. "It wasn't a surprise or shock," he said. "It was more of a confirmation. If it had been cancer, that would have been more shocking." His mom would not have tested for Huntington's disease on her own, but the family was concerned about her declining health. "When she got the test result," Rob said, "she mentally shut down. She's in denial of the whole disease, while the rest of the family is quite proactive."

His mom's experience highlights the need for more awareness among healthcare practitioners. "I understand they cannot know everything about every disease, but there's still a lot of harm being done," Rob said. He described what happened when his family realized his mom needed to move to a long-term care facility. Rob's mom had started injuring herself when trying to perform everyday tasks, like cutting herself when trying to peel a potato. Rob's dad knew she needed more care than he could provide, so they met with her general practitioner (GP) to start the process of transitioning to long-term care.

The GP knew Rob's mom had Huntington's disease, so Rob was surprised by the doctor's response. "The GP said, and I kid you not, 'We should not do anything. One of these days, she will fall down the stairs. She will break her leg, and when she's in the hospital, we can take her out of the house without any hassle.' Those were literally his words," Rob said. This doctor retired soon after this conversation, and the new GP immediately recognized that Rob's mom needed long-term care. This doctor started the necessary paperwork after meeting her just once, and within half a year, Rob's mom moved to the care home where she still lives today.

Rob feels lucky to live in the Netherlands, where there is a well-organized network of care homes specializing in HD care. These care homes communicate with each other about best practices, and they have social workers who work with HD families. Rob's mom is on the waiting list for one of these specialized facilities, but she is content in her current care home. "We decided not to move her as long as she's happy where she is," he said. "If the care demand becomes too high for that care home, then she can move. That's a sort of peace of mind that we have."

Soon after his mom's diagnosis, Rob reached out to a genetic center to start the testing process. During the counseling phase, however, Rob realized he was too preoccupied with his mom's diagnosis to get his own result, so he paused the process. He resumed the process a year or two later when his leg started twitching at night and he became convinced he had Huntington's disease. "I tested positive for Huntington's," he said, "and the twitchy leg disappeared." He now knows that he gets restless legs when he is under stress.

For Rob, one of the hardest parts of belonging to an HD family is losing somebody over a prolonged period. "I think of how my mother was before she became really sick. That person is no longer there, and that's not nice to see," he said. "That is quite an understatement, obviously. Seeing your aunt, and your grandmother, and all the struggle that your family members have with the kids and the mortgages – that can be painful at times. Most of the time, I cope with it quite well, but sometimes, it just hits you. So that's tough." Another downside is seeing the same progression in friends from the HD community. "There are people who were okay last year. This year, they cannot function properly anymore. You lose a lot of people."

To cope with Huntington's disease, Rob finds it helpful to talk with others and write about his experiences. "I talk to roughly everybody about this," he said. "I'm quite an open book in that respect. There's no shame in having this disease. You always hear that when people get this kind of bad news, they change their whole lives. I've never done that. I've stayed on my own path. When I got my own positive test result, that slowly became part of me. It didn't change me as a person. I've always done volunteering, but mainly with the sports club. Now, I volunteer for a patient organization. It doesn't feel like I'm doing anything else – it's just the cause is different. I'm just being me."

While Rob is comfortable talking about any HD-related topic, he was once asked a question that took him aback. He was doing an interview for a documentary about genetic diseases. When Rob mentioned that he and his wife were going through IVF to conceive an HD-free child, the interviewer asked what would happen if Rob became symptomatic soon after having a baby. Was Rob afraid of how that would affect his child? "And honestly," Rob said, "until that moment, I had not given that one second of thought. I always assumed we have late onset, so my son will be 15 to 20." However, Rob knows he could have symptom onset earlier than his mother. "Either I actively ignored that fact or… I don't know…"

Rob is in his early 40s, and he knows his life would look different if he was already symptomatic. "We have a baby boy now," he said. "He's quite a character. It is the best thing that has happened so far in my life. I'm still healthy. If I were symptomatic, I don't think we would have a family." The interviewer's question got Rob thinking, though, so he set up the Netherlands' equivalent of an advanced directive to protect his son. "Before you become unfit, you can put your decisions on paper and get it official," he said. "In that sense, I know how to prevent negative things from happening to my son. But of course, deep down in my heart,

I know that doesn't mean that he won't be hurt by the fact that his father will get sick and die. I don't have a solution for that. It will be an incredibly sad moment when they tell me, 'You've become symptomatic, and now is the moment a decline has started.' If that happens in the next year or so, that will be horrible."

Rob works for a startup company that develops gene therapies for Huntington's disease and ALS. As a senior scientist, he develops methods to measure whether potential gene therapies treat what they are meant to treat on the molecular level. He is involved in the company's research design process through each stage, starting at the molecular level, moving to animal models, and eventually to human clinical trials. This involves answering questions such as: What should be measured and how? What is needed to decide readiness to move to the next stage? How should a potential treatment be administered? What should patient involvement look like?

The collaborative nature of HD research is invaluable to Rob. When designing a clinical trial, he and his colleagues reach out to the CHDI Foundation and other HD networks to get feedback. They all share information about what they have tried, what has or has not worked, and how to avoid mistakes. The high volume of HD research increases the likelihood of success down the road. "People always want results quickly, but clinical trials and drug development take years and years to get somewhere," Rob said. "For Huntington's, there are many companies working on it. If one fails, you want to have five that are safely behind it, and the next one, and then the next one. You don't want to rely on one company because if it fails, it'll take another 15 years to get one step further."

In his own work, Rob sees that the HD research community is more organized and has more participation from patients than he sees with other diseases. He has been pleasantly surprised at how easy it has been to fill spots for HD clinical trials. A recent phase 3 clinical trial from Roche quickly filled 1,000 slots. "It shows you a bit about the HD community," he said. "They are organized through all the networks: HDSA, the Canadians, the European Huntington Association. There are

Enroll-HD sites all over the globe, so we have a database of more than 20,000 people to identify candidates who are a potential fit for a trial. That's impressive." This is quite different from the work Rob has done with ALS. "I see how much more effort it takes and how much more it costs on the ALS side versus the Huntington's side," he said. "For HD, if you want biological samples, you can file a request to Enroll-HD. You have one central point where you can get your information."

Rob thinks this is a unique moment in HD history because of the high volume of research in progress. Ninety percent of all clinical trials are unsuccessful, but even failed trials contribute to forward movement of the field. When the high-profile Roche trial was halted, there was significant disappointment in the HD community, but Rob continues to be optimistic. "There's so much data behind such a trial that it's difficult to understand it all. I was at a Huntington's conference in Boston, and I heard pharmaceutical companies talking about what they've learned from these failures. It's impressive. As a scientist, it makes me happy," he said. "As a patient, I'm not happy. But as a scientist, I'm like, wow – what a wealth of information."

Like many others in the HD community, Rob finds hope in research. "I'm a glass-half-full kind of person," he said. "Just the fact that there are so many companies working on it makes me hopeful. I'm not saying that in five years we will have something, but it gets closer and closer all the time. I'm doubtful something will be available in my lifetime, but I'm sure there will be some treatment available for the next generation." Rob strongly encourages the HD community to get involved in research, whether that is taking part in clinical trials, Enroll-HD, surveys, or other observational studies. Clinical trial participation is not risk-free, nor does it guarantee a medical benefit, but many who take part in research find it gives them purpose and motivation. "I understand why people do it. But behind that selfish reasoning, there is quite a philanthropic thing," Rob said. "They contribute so much that they are probably not even aware of. They do a lot of good for the community."

Rob shared an example from a recent HD meeting where Emmy award-winning journalist, Charles Sabine, who is gene positive, talked about donating cerebral spinal fluid for HD research years ago. That sample is still used in studies today. "Research takes time," Rob said, "but you can donate some blood now, and maybe in 10 or 15 years, that blood will help us understand the disease better. It doesn't cost you much, but it can give us a lot. The power is in the numbers – the more people participate, the better information we can get. If you have an opportunity to take part, it's always great to do it."

Incorporating the patient voice

The Huntington's Disease Coalition for Patient Engagement (HD-COPE) and the Huntington's Disease Community Advisory Board (HD-CAB) are coalitions of HD community members who share the realities of living with Huntington's disease with industry partners, including researchers, pharmaceutical companies, regulators, and policymakers. Their perspectives provide insight into the challenges of participating in research as well as what HD patients are willing to risk or tolerate in return for a chance to help find treatments. As a member of HD-COPE, Jenna recognizes the importance of giving the HD community a voice in clinical research, and she hopes the groups' efforts will benefit her family and others one day.

Jenna is a teacher in the greater Toronto area and a mother to two young girls. She knew nothing about Huntington's disease when her mom started exhibiting strange behavioral symptoms more than a decade ago. Jenna's family always found an explanation for her mom's irrationality, irritability, and physical and verbal aggression. "A lot of the behavioral changes initially had to do with her relationship with my father," Jenna said. "We attributed it to poor communication in my parents' marriage." It also made sense that Jenna's mom struggled when she entered menopause and when two close loved ones died. Their family doctor concluded Jenna's mom had depression even though medication and therapy didn't help.

Jenna was alarmed when she watched an episode of the television show, *Breaking Bad*, in which the main character, Walter White, described his father's HD symptoms. His description sounded all too familiar. "I knew right away that was what she had," Jenna said. "Despite not having any sort of psychosis, she had all the symptoms. We also had family members who had involuntary movements." Jenna's mom had always described her family as fidgety people. Jenna was certain she had the answer to what had been a decade-long journey to make sense of her mom's symptoms. Their family doctor, however, was dismissive. Instead of referring Jenna's mom for genetic testing, he suggested cognitive behavioral therapy, long walks, and more communication with Jenna's dad. "He didn't have background knowledge about HD, and he just couldn't wrap his mind around the fact that I was coming to him with a possible diagnosis," Jenna said.

With help from a social worker at the Huntington Society of Canada, Jenna's mom connected with a genetic counselor and received an HD diagnosis. When Jenna told her aunt about her mom's HD diagnosis, Jenna learned that her uncle tested positive five years earlier but didn't disclose it to the rest of the family. Her aunt and uncle wanted to protect family members from the news. "In those five years," Jenna said, "my brother had children. He could have had children a different way had he known he was at risk. It is an immense amount of pressure and guilt for parents to know they could have passed it on. Now everyone knows we have a genetic disease in our family and can make informed choices about the future."

Jenna sought out genetic testing about a year after her mom's diagnosis because she and her partner were thinking of having children. Jenna was grateful when she tested negative, but when she received her result, she felt, "Numb. Just numb. Unbelievable. I had convinced myself that I carried the gene." Jenna isn't sure how many of her at-risk family members have gone through genetic testing. "My mom has three siblings," she said. "Between the siblings there are 10 kids – my cousins. To my knowledge, only a few of us have done genetic testing. Many have either done genetic testing and not disclosed it or haven't done testing and have gone on to have children. We've got another generation of kids at risk. We need a treatment."

Jenna's mom has changed considerably over the years. As Jenna described it, "It's like I'm standing on a dock, and there's a boat sailing off in the distance and getting harder to see. I'm left with who she is now – a shell of who she once was. I hold on so dearly to my memories, and I struggle with the fact that she's been symptomatic for half my life." Jenna spoke about what her mom was like when Jenna was a kid. Her mom made beautiful gift baskets for every birthday and holiday and planned lots of activities during school breaks. "I try to take those things I love the most and incorporate them into my own life as a mother. She was so lovely," Jenna said. "I'm in a perpetual state of grief. I'm grieving what's happened, and I'm grieving what I anticipate is going to happen. I find it difficult."

Since her mom's diagnosis, Jenna has played a large role in caring for her mom and supporting her dad. Helping her parents, working full-time, and caring for her young daughters took a toll on Jenna. She reached a breaking point when her mom had three major falls that resulted in more than 10 fractures and multiple hospital stays. Jenna took time off work and reached out to a social worker. "She helped me recognize just how much I was taking on and the impact it was having on me. It wasn't sustainable," Jenna said. Jenna's mom eventually moved to a long-term care facility, a move that has been beneficial to Jenna's mom and the rest of the family.

Jenna feels a strong sense of commitment to the HD community, so she has taken on several volunteer roles. "I have the skillset, the motivation, and the initiative. It would be a waste to not channel it into patient advocacy," she said. After getting involved in youth programming and youth mentorship with the Huntington Society of Canada, Jenna became a project coordinator with HDYO and worked to launch the Youth and Young Adult Mentorship Program in partnership with HDSA.

Jenna talked about the importance of sharing patient perspectives with industry partners through her work as a member of HD-COPE. "All of them indicated it was beneficial to have an organization like HD-COPE ready and available to meet with them," Jenna said. "Our group had a good understanding of the clinical trial process. We'd been trained in key terminology and the different processes that take place, and we had training on policies in different parts of the world. And then we were given a more specialized explanation of the science behind all the different therapies the companies were developing."

It is important for industry partners to understand the physical, cognitive, and emotional impacts of Huntington's disease on everyone involved. To convey the lived experience of Huntington's disease, HD-COPE members represent a variety of roles, including family caregivers and people who are at risk, gene positive, and gene negative. Industry partners are knowledgeable about Huntington's disease, but Jenna thinks their interactions with HD-COPE have increased their understanding. "It's not until they're in a room with 20 family members that they see how different it is from one person to the next and the extremes that you can have," she said. "You can have one person with subtle involuntary movements that aren't problematic, and another with ballistic chorea that's completely debilitating."

When members of HD-COPE provide feedback on clinical trial design, industry partners are interested in answers to questions like: What do you think of our trial design? What do you think of these assessments? What about this method of administering medication? Where is it important to have caregiver input? "We would relate our lived experience and what we would anticipate could happen in those scenarios," Jenna said. "I would talk about having a young family and wanting my mom to participate in clinical trials, but I can't take three days off work every two months to bring her to the clinical trial. It's overwhelming – the costs that are associated with that, the length of appointment visits, and the logistics around planning and organizing to attend visits, in addition to managing the logistics of having a young family."

HD-CAB is a similar patient advocacy group. It was created in 2021 to give a voice to HD community members who often do not have a seat at the table, including people from countries outside North America, young adults, and HD community members who are at risk, presymptomatic, or in the prodromal stage (i.e., experiencing early symptoms but not yet symptomatic enough to receive a clinical diagnosis). In addition to sharing their experiences with industry partners, members of HD-CAB also receive education on how research moves from the laboratory to clinical trials to becoming a drug or therapy available to patients. "I'm happy to see this starting," Jenna said. "I believe that the more young people understand the clinical trial process and what it means to be involved, the more they will be informed and able to encourage their loved ones to get involved."

Jenna is a strong proponent of getting tested for Huntington's disease to become eligible for clinical trials, and yet she knows how big of an ask that is. Without a cure or treatment, the percentage of people who go through predictive genetic testing remains low. Jenna's not sure she would have been ready to deal with a positive test result herself. "When I walked out of the hospital," she said, "I thought, I will *never* encourage someone to do what I just went through. It's contradictory because I'm saying we need people to do genetic testing so they can participate in clinical trials so we can find treatments. But I remember thinking I could *never* live through that again or wish that upon anyone."

Many organizations, including those Jenna has worked with, have begun considering the importance of accessibility, affordability, and availability of any drugs that might eventually come on the market to treat Huntington's disease. If a future treatment needs to be administered by lumbar injection, for example, the cost may be high, and accessibility to treatment sites may be low. Jenna is glad to see these conversations taking place now because addressing these issues will be central to the success of any future treatments.

After several years of promoting the patient voice, Jenna is surprised there hasn't been an even greater emphasis on patient involvement. "One thing I've noticed is that incorporating the patients' voice into any conversation about healthcare is important, whether it be drug policy that is dictated by the government, or development of clinical trials, or regulatory processes," she said. "Patient involvement is so important, so valuable, and it seems like it should be the place to start rather than an afterthought."

HD-COPE members are often asked what they see as the most pressing HD issues that need to be addressed. For Jenna and her family, managing her mom's behavioral symptoms has been the biggest challenge. For her gene-positive friend, however, the most pressing thing is extending the number of high-quality years she'll get to spend with her young children. "She's getting to the point where her best years are behind her. So, to have a drug that would extend those good-quality years is important," Jenna said. "That's powerful. That really is it. It's not about chorea or behavior or emotions. People need better, longer, quality of life."

What does it mean to have hope in research? To me, it means trusting scientists will continue to expand our knowledge about Huntington's disease and identify innovative ways to interrupt its progression. It also means trusting that it won't be long before receiving an HD diagnosis no longer signals a patient's decline, but instead opens doors for a patient to gain access to disease-modifying treatments. For now, members of the HD community are left wondering how much our loved ones will decline and how many more people will die from Huntington's disease before researchers reach these lofty goals.

Research relies on participation by members of the HD community, something many people are willing to do. Participating in research at any level – surveys, observational studies, or clinical trials – is an important and meaningful contribution to improving our understanding of Huntington's disease. Being selected for a clinical trial that might identify the next step toward treating or curing this disease is like winning the lottery. Participation in most clinical trials, however, requires patients to have a clinical diagnosis. This typically doesn't happen until chorea is present, which is after brain atrophy and early cognitive and behavioral symptoms are well underway. By then, HD patients have already experienced irreversible changes.

Ultimately, members of the HD community want a safe and effective way to stop the progression of Huntington's disease before the neurodegenerative process begins – to prevent disease altogether. Getting there will take many more research studies and clinical trials, a lot of time and funding, and continued participation by the HD community. But it will also require a better grasp of early disease progression to unlock opportunities for presymptomatic and prodromal patients to participate in clinical research. Focusing research on this early period is critical to the goal of preventing disease rather than treating symptoms after disease progression has already begun.

When I think about having hope in research, it's about much more than scientific progress. The heart of my hope lies in looking ahead to a time when HD families can make plans for a longer and healthier future with our loved ones. There is no time to waste.

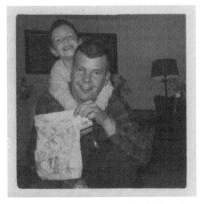

Research is key to a future in which Huntington's disease can be delayed, slowed, or prevented so we have more quality time with our loved ones.

RESOURCES

Research Updates

Most HD organizations communicate research findings to their followers on social media, and the following provide articles and/or webinars that explain research findings to nonscientists: *HD Buzz* provides easy-to-understand articles; the Hereditary Disease Foundation hosts a research webinar series; and the Huntington Study Group produces a semiannual research review called, *HD Insights*.

Patient Registries

Patient registries gather observational data that inform HD research, and some are used to recruit participants for HD research studies. Enroll-HD (CHDI Foundation), RARE-X (HDSA and HD Reach), and myHDstory (Huntington Study Group) are international registries, and the Map-HD Registry (HDNA) is an Australian registry. In addition, JOIN-HD (HDYO) serves as an international patient registry for Juvenile Huntington's disease.

Clinical Trials

To learn about clinical trials, contact your national HD organization. In addition, two databases provide information about upcoming, ongoing, and completed clinical trials: HD Trial Finder (HDSA) and ClinicalTrials.gov (National Institutes of Health). Both are international in scope. If you live in the United States or Canada, HD Genetics can connect you with opportunities to participate in clinical and observational research.

Patient Advocacy Organizations

To learn more about efforts to incorporate the patient voice into the research process, check out the Huntington's Disease Community Advisory Board (HD-CAB) and the Huntington's Disease Coalition for Patient Engagement (HD-COPE).

HOPE AND MEANING

Having hope in something, big or small, is a fundamental part of life. Hope can take on different forms like purpose, a positive outlook, or faith. This is the stuff that helps us get up every day – the stuff that pulls us through the hard times and keeps us moving forward. And yet, *hope* can be a problematic word. There are times when it can feel impossible for HD families to find their hope, like when HD symptoms are severe, crises arise, or a major research study fails. When others tell us we just need to have hope, it falls flat because hope doesn't spring to life spontaneously; it has to originate somewhere. Despite the complexities that come with it, *hope* is a topic I wanted to explore.

In my conversations with the HD community, I didn't ask about hope so I could show how resilient this community is, though there is no better word to describe the grit people show when facing this disease. I didn't ask about hope so I could create a list of things the HD community can be grateful for, even though people mentioned many things they've gained by living in the HD world. I knew that asking about hope might feel like a strange question given the subject matter, but I truly wanted to know what gives members of the HD community hope. Seeking answers to this question seemed fundamental to understanding how people face each day given the challenges presented by Huntington's disease. I wanted honest answers, and I got them.

The people I spoke with find hope in obvious things like researchers finding a treatment or cure, preventing the disease from passing to the next generation, or wishing a loved one won't have to suffer too much for too long. As people talked about hope, they also talked about what they find meaningful in their lives. They mentioned things like contributing to a better life for others, appreciating the good things in life, raising awareness, or finding ways to live independently as long as possible. I learned that many people actively create their own livable life in which hope and meaning become lifelines. Ultimately, they find hope and meaning in knowing and being known by loved ones, connecting with others, and making a difference.

Knowing each other

One of the biggest things Huntington's disease takes away is our ability to know each other. As people with the disease experience cognitive losses, behavioral changes, and impaired speech, it becomes harder for them to communicate effectively and for loved ones to recognize them as the person they were before symptom onset. In addition, our loved ones with Huntington's disease pass away when they are much too young and often after a significant period of decline. Our ability to interact with and know each other diminishes, and our time together is too short.

Once I learned we are an HD family, I realized I never truly knew my dad. For me, this is one of the saddest parts of my own HD story. I now know that a big piece of my life is missing because the inaccessible and difficult father I thought I knew was a manifestation of his HD symptoms. I didn't get to have a relationship with the father I could have had – the father I should have had. It would have meant so much to me to have had a chance to know what he was really like and for him to have

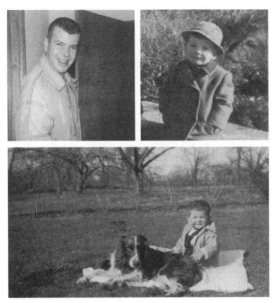

When I visited my dad's hometown, I gained a better understanding of what his life was like long before he developed Huntington's disease.

had a chance to know me as an adult.

My dad's been gone a long time now. As much as I wish I could, I cannot go back in time and get to know what he was like before his symptoms began. All I can do is piece together tidbits of his life. When I was a teenager and young adult, my dad didn't talk much or share a lot, so most of what I know about his childhood comes from long-ago conversations with my grandma and my aunt's stories. My aunt wrote about family gatherings and the Connecticut house she and my dad grew up in. She wrote about the trouble they used to get into, spending time at the beach, and exploring the woods around their house. These stories give me a small peek into my dad's childhood, but I'm so glad I didn't leave it at that.

Several months after I started my conversations with the HD community, I visited places tied to my dad's childhood. There is something about being in a place that fills gaps in your knowledge you didn't even know were there. By immersing myself in places central to my dad's upbringing, I gained a deeper understanding of who he was. As I explored his hometown and saw his grandparents' homes, my vision of his childhood became rooted in my senses. I heard the bugs and birds in the trees and the water moving along the brooks. I noticed the light shimmering through the autumn-tinged leaves overhead. I smelled the sea air as I walked on the beach and climbed on the same rocks he climbed on all those years ago.

As I walked through his childhood home and explored the places he loved, his childhood seemed almost idyllic. I'm grateful for that. There's only so much I can learn about my dad now that he's gone, but even the small things I piece together help me know him a little better. They add depth to the person I knew when I was a young adult and help me imagine what he was like as a little boy and young man. These things help me feel more connected to him and make me wish even more that I could have known him better.

Now, I look for ways to continue to know my brother. Our interactions change as my brother's symptoms progress, and connecting with him takes more effort than it used to. We can no longer have easy casual conversations, so I ask my brother questions about things from the past that I think his kids might be interested in knowing about him. I hope this gives them insight into his pre-HD life. My brother replies with brief responses – "That's right!" or "I did!" – so most of the information comes from my questions rather than his answers. Still, sharing stories with him is part of maintaining our connection and reminding my brother that he is worth knowing. He still has a story to tell, even if he needs help telling it.

As I transcribed my conversations with the HD community, I realized I was listening to many people in their own pre-HD life, or maybe even in the earliest stages of their disease. I recorded their voices and their stories at a time when they could easily share their thoughts. They expressed their wishes, their fears, their love for their families. They talked about their hopes for the future and what the disease has taken from them and their families. Those who are gene positive will change considerably in the next 10, 20, or 30 years. When they enter the last stage of their disease, their families will think back and wish they could remember what they were like or wish they had known them better before symptoms began.

HD families know their lives will change dramatically as their loved ones progress through their disease. Knowing what lies ahead, many people actively create a bank of memories so one day they can look back and remember positive times together. Creating and maintaining these shared experiences and connections is a meaningful act because time together is limited. As symptoms progress, it becomes important to find new ways to connect with and know our loved ones who have Huntington's disease so we can continue this act of knowing and being known by each other.

One gene-positive *Livable Lives* storyteller makes scrapbooks for each phase of her life. When she has children one day, she plans to use the scrapbooks to tell them about her life. Later, when she's bedridden and no longer able to communicate, her family can use the scrapbooks to remind her of adventures from her youth. She's only 24, but she's already thinking about how to connect with her family when she's in the late stage of her disease. She's not alone. Lily is another *Livable Lives* storyteller who thanked me for the opportunity to record her story so she can share it with her son, Gabe, one day. Lily, who is gene positive, is grateful she was young when Gabe was born so she'll have more time to know him – and he'll have more time to know her – before her symptoms progress.

We were joined by Lily's younger half-sister, Ella, who is at risk. Lily is eight years older than Ella, and it was easy to see they are close. The sisters can trace their HD roots to their maternal great-grandfather. He was never diagnosed with Huntington's disease, but in hindsight he had classic symptoms. Their grandmother and aunt both passed away from Huntington's disease, but their uncle has not been tested and has never developed symptoms.

Their mom was initially diagnosed with postpartum depression after Ella was born, but her depression didn't subside, and other HD symptoms appeared. "It was this slow progression into the disease," said Lily. Later, things became especially difficult for their family when their mom started having more emotional and psychiatric symptoms, including hallucinations. "The psychiatric symptoms were harder on our family than the physical stuff," said Lily. When their mom's symptoms became very pronounced and she refused to take medication, she was admitted to the state hospital and both girls were removed from the home.

For the next several years, Lily and Ella moved between their grandfather's home and their uncle's home. Luckily, medication made a world of difference for their mom. "It was like night and day," said Lily. Eventually, Ella and their mom went to live with Ella's dad. When their mom needed more care than Ella and her dad could provide at home, their mom moved to a nursing home, where she now receives hospice care.

Because of their age difference, Lily and Ella each saw different stages of their mom's disease. Lily had the chance to know their mom before symptom onset. Their mom was a nurse who was physically active and rode her bike everywhere. Lily has vague memories of these early years, but old family pictures, in which their mom often looks happy, help fill in the gaps. Ella lived with their mom when symptoms were at their worst. "She was pretty different at different stages," Ella said. "Her personality changed a lot."

Ella recalled many good memories of her mom. "When I was little, she loved caring for me," Ella said. "She was always there when I was sick, giving me a cool rag for a fever, or giving me medicine." Ella has fond memories of family trips, and she likes hearing her family and her mom's friends recount stories about her mom as a young woman. She was a very caring person who was always helping people.

When Ella was a college student, she was interested in biology, but she didn't think she would pursue an MD or PhD degree because there might not be enough time to pay off college debt and enjoy a long career if she were to develop Huntington's disease. So, she hoped to find a science career that would suit her needs regardless of what her gene status is. By the time she finished her bachelor's degree, Ella's view of Huntington's disease had changed considerably. "At some point," she realized, "even if it is important to consider for future planning, I don't have to let HD dictate every part of my life." She now feels like she can make plans despite the uncertainty introduced by Huntington's disease. "Nothing's guaranteed," she said. Ella is now applying for a PhD program and taking things one step at a time.

Ella's ability to share her experiences with Huntington's disease has also changed. She used to be uncomfortable telling friends about her mom until she had known them for a long time. Now, Ella is more involved in the HD community, and she is also a Young Adult Rare Representative with the EveryLife Foundation for Rare Diseases. She interacts with people from other disease communities, and she is learning how to advocate for the rare disease community at-large. This involvement has made her much more at ease with sharing her own story. "Growing up, I'd stay quiet about a lot of things," she said. "That was the safer route for me, but I realized not being able to feel like myself with other people was causing me a lot of harm. Having that freedom to share more about myself and how this impacts me has been helpful. It takes time to practice that skill to be open with people. Also, I want to make a difference for the community."

Ella is comfortable being at risk, but Lily found it exhausting, so she sought out genetic testing in 2019. A romantic relationship had just ended, so Lily thought things couldn't get worse. "You hold onto that little piece of hope. You're going to have a cloud over your head, regardless, but if it came back negative, then I could live my life," Lily said. "I knew it was going to be positive, and I prepared myself for that, but finding out made it certain. I swore I was ready, but I probably could have waited a little bit."

Lily was a teenager when she had Gabe, and she dreamed of having a big family someday. After testing positive, though, dating was challenging. Some guys were able to accept that she was a single mom but unable to accept a future that included Huntington's disease. Lily is now in a relationship that has lasted several years. "I'm comfortable and content in my life," she said. "I have a healthy relationship and things I didn't have before. So, I found out this horrible thing, but at the same time, some good things have found their way in."

Even so, Lily thinks it's harder to know that she is gene positive than it was to be at risk. "You never have relief either way," she said. "You still have other people in your family that could have it, but at least I can start planning things. I'm still young. I still have a lot of time, but it does dictate a lot of my choices." Lily's mixed feelings after testing positive influenced Ella's decision to remain at risk. Ella also feels like she is gene positive. "Either way," Ella said, "it won't necessarily be a good outcome. Lily tested positive, so there's always going to be HD in my life."

Lily can already feel herself changing. She notices changes in her personality, she forgets things, and she trips easily. She can't get away from the thought that these are approaching signs of Huntington's disease, especially when she finds it difficult to complete a task. "I'm constantly thinking in the back of my head that that's the disease," she said. "Sometimes, I just don't feel the same, and that is so scary." To calm her frustration when things don't go right, she tells herself over and over that her disease onset hasn't started yet.

Now that Lily knows she's gene positive, she understands her mother in a way she never did before. She always admired her mom's efforts to live a full life. "I understand some of the pain and emotions that were a big part of her life," Lily said. "It's easier to understand when you're living it day-to-day. You realize that many people don't have that desire to live their life. They have all this healthy life, but they waste it." For now, Lily tries to put her worries on the back burner and focus on living in the present. She succeeds most of the time, but it's hard to avoid those thoughts when she visits her mom.

Lily doesn't want Gabe to fear Huntington's disease, so she takes him to visit his grandma at the nursing home regularly. Lily answers his questions after these visits, but she hasn't told him specifics about the disease or shared that she's gene positive. Lily struggles with how and when to share these things with Gabe because she wants him to live life freely. For now, telling him about the disease a little at a time feels like enough. "One day, I will have those conversations, but it is hard to know when a good time is," she said. "He's 11 now. I don't want to put that thought into his head until he's mature enough to understand and cope with it. I don't know why I've been so guarded with him. I think I just want him to be a kid. My biggest fear is him having it, which I never talk about. That's obviously worse than having it myself."

Lily feels fortunate she was young when Gabe was born so she'll have more time with him before her disease progresses too far. "It's not just my future I'm worried about – it's his," she said. "When I saw this opportunity to share my story, I honestly broke down in tears. Having something for him to look back on to understand the things that we often don't talk about – no matter how big or small – means an awful lot. It's something I wish I had for our mom."

Lily finds hope in feeling like the people she cares about are going to be okay. "My sister has this amazing career path ahead of her, and I'm in a healthy relationship now that allows me to breathe," she said. "We have a support system within our family – not many people can say that. If anything were to happen, I know Gabe's in good hands; everyone's in good hands." Lily finds comfort in knowing that Gabe will be grown up by the time her disease progresses to a more advanced stage. "Hopefully, by that point, he'll be more capable of understanding, more capable of coping. Knowing that I can see a lot of his life, too, gives me a little bit of hope."

Connecting with others

Members of the HD community find hope and meaning in connecting with each other. HD conventions, support groups, and youth camps are instrumental in helping us feel like we don't have to face this life alone. When we gather together, we can finally talk openly about our experiences. We don't have to explain the complexities of Huntington's disease as we share our stories, and we can connect with people we can turn to when we have questions or concerns. In a small amount of time, these connections can develop into an extended family. I don't know if this is a worldwide phenomenon, but many people in North America refer to this chosen HD family as their *Ohana*.

When things were difficult with my dad, and later when we learned we are an HD family, it was easy to feel like no one would understand what my family was facing. I had people around me who cared about me, but they weren't grappling with the same struggles and questions I was. My feelings of isolation came from a lack of shared experience, not a lack of caring. When I went to my first HD support group, I met people who had had experiences like my own. They were strangers, and yet I immediately knew they offered a safe space to explore how I felt. These connections provided my first glimmer of hope that I was going to be okay.

Years later, when I went to my first national HD convention and found myself in the presence of hundreds of people impacted by Huntington's disease, I felt a sense of ease I don't think I had ever experienced before. I've spent much of my life feeling like my experiences set me apart, so feeling like I was one-among-many stripped away many of the barriers I've built up over time to protect myself. I felt at home.

Many of the people I spoke with talked about attending HD youth camps that transformed their perception of Huntington's disease and made them feel like they finally had a supportive community where they belonged. When I had the opportunity to volunteer at one of these camps, I jumped at the chance. The experience was exactly what people had talked about. Over the course of a few days, campers transformed from a group of strangers into a solid base of support they will carry with them into their everyday lives.

These connections provide hope and meaning by creating a sense of belonging that we all need and crave. While conventions, camps, and support groups provide opportunities to meet members of the HD community, they are not the only ways to connect with others. It's possible to create our own opportunities to connect with others. While creating community is challenging when you're a member of a rare disease community, the benefits of doing so can be significant. Connecting with others provides a home, a safe space, and comfort when it's needed most. Mackenzie Remillard is a gene-negative young man from Canada who learned about creating community from his father. Hope is what drives him to connect with and advocate for the HD community.

Mackenzie always knew Huntington's disease was in his family. His grandfather died of Huntington's disease before he was born, and he remembers when his aunt was in the late stage of the disease. Mackenzie's mom tested positive for Huntington's disease soon after predictive genetic testing became available in the 1990s but long before she had symptoms. When Mackenzie's parents met, his mom was open about her positive gene status, and Mackenzie's dad wasn't scared away. Mackenzie didn't know his mom was gene positive until she started showing symptoms when he was 10 years old.

Mackenzie grew up watching his cousins care for their mom. He knew it was going to be hard to see his mom go through the same thing as his aunt, but he didn't completely understand the extent of it. His cousins hadn't talked much about what it was like to care for their mom, so Mackenzie assumed he and his family would be able to continue with their everyday lives. "I knew it would be a burden on my family, but I didn't think it would be as much a part of my life as it is," he said. "I expected it to be hard, but not this hard."

While his family talked openly about Huntington's disease, Mackenzie was reluctant to share with people outside his family. He was a quiet kid and had a lot of anxiety. He's glad he grew up in a small town with supportive friends who knew his mom had Huntington's disease, and he appreciated that they would ask how she was doing. "I got pretty lucky with the people I was surrounded by and the way my family was," he said.

Mackenzie's mom's symptoms began with small twitches in her hands and feet and progressed slowly at first. Now, her symptoms are hard to miss. "Everyone notices when she's in the room because she's at the point she seems like she's drunk, but she's not," Mackenzie said.

"Her speech is slurred, and she has bad balance and forgets words." Mackenzie has also noticed a change in his mom's hugs. "I've hugged enough people in the HD community that I'm starting to see that progress into her hug," he said. "It's like stopping motions – more like a chorea-movement hug." Mackenzie's mom struggles with the emotional symptoms of Huntington's disease, but her current mix of medications is working well. She's generally happy and only has infrequent bouts of anger. She's still able to enjoy life and spends her days doing things she likes. "My family has two dogs and three cats," Mackenzie said, "so she spends her day cuddling with all of them."

Mackenzie used to play a large role in helping his mom during outbursts. "I've heard from other families with similar experiences that there's always one person in the family that's able to calm down the person with HD," he said. "That person was me. I was always a mediator between my mom and whomever she was having an argument with." That often meant inserting himself into arguments between his mom and his dad or sister. If things got heated while he was away, arguments could last for hours until he returned home and helped his mom settle. "It was hard for me personally," he said. "I'm still trying to find a way to take some of that weight off."

Huntington's disease has affected family relationships in other ways as well. "Growing up, me and my mom were attached at the hip," Mackenzie said. "It's hard to grieve that I'm losing my mom even though she's still alive. She no longer fits the average role of a mother. We take care of her, and at times it feels as if I'm her parent." Mackenzie's parents' relationship has also changed as his mom has needed more care. His dad now thinks of his mom as more of a best friend than a spouse. "He still loves her, but it's a different kind of love," Mackenzie said. "We're losing the person that she was." Mackenzie knows they will experience another kind of loss when his mom eventually passes away, so he cherishes the time he has with her and holds on to memories of what she used to be like.

Three youth mentors from the HD community have played an important role in helping Mackenzie cope with his mom's illness, normal teen troubles, and the testing process. One of the mentors is also gene negative and understands Mackenzie's struggle to move forward after learning his gene status. Mackenzie had planned his life around developing Huntington's disease one day, so it's hard to envision a gene-negative version of his future. It's difficult to be happy when he's worried about his gene-positive friends.

Mackenzie is glad he's had a chance to connect with and learn from others who are gene negative. He's met several who went through a period of feeling disconnected from the HD community after testing and before becoming advocates for family and friends who are at risk or gene positive. "I'm gene negative, so I can advocate for my friends who are positive," Mackenzie said. "Twenty years from now, most of them are going to have symptoms. They're going to need someone to advocate for them, and I want that to be me." Mackenzie now has a new direction and purpose and is inspired to be more involved in the HD community.

Growing up, Mackenzie watched his dad create an environment in which their family did not have to feel alone. When the family moved to a small town with a population of 1,200, they found that few people knew about Huntington's disease. Mackenzie's dad went door-to-door to tell people about Mackenzie's gene-positive mom and raise money for an annual Indy Go-Kart fundraiser that supports the local chapter of the Huntington Society of Canada (HSC). Mackenzie's dad actively built a supportive community for his family by educating people about Huntington's disease. His dad also encouraged the family to talk openly. Over time, residents came to know Mackenzie's family and gained an understanding of Huntington's disease.

Mackenzie is following in his father's footsteps by actively cultivating his own community. He is involved in a wide variety of HD outreach and education activities. He regularly attends national conferences for the HSC as well as youth events and camps, and he serves on several boards. He's an active fundraiser, a trained youth mentor with HSC, and an HDYO ambassador. Mackenzie knows getting involved in the HD community can be daunting, but he's gained a lot from his experiences. "It's shaped the person I am today through the connections I've made," he said. "I sometimes say, 'It's terrible I got the chance to meet you because of this disease,' but I'm so thankful because they're all great people, and they all understand."

While Mackenzie was shy when he was younger, he is now comfortable talking about all aspects of Huntington's disease, even his own anxiety and depression. "Growing up," he said, "I was a shy kid who held everything in. I slowly started to self-destruct at grade eight or nine because I was dealing with all these big things. They were piling up. Then I realized that when I share my story about Huntington's, it's like letting it off my shoulders a little bit. And maybe it can help other people as well, so I became an open book."

Now that Mackenzie openly shares his HD story, his childhood friends have a better sense of what his home life was like growing up. While they knew his mom had Huntington's disease, they didn't know how that affected Mackenzie's mental health. They didn't see the day-to-day struggles that take place in an HD family. Mackenzie's friends thought he was coping well, but he was struggling. Mackenzie thinks his experience helps him understand others better, and he no longer assumes that others aren't facing their own challenges.

Mackenzie's view of Huntington's disease has changed considerably over time. When his mom was first diagnosed, his only experience was his aunt's later stages of the disease. He focused on his mom's future, which was frightening. Getting involved in the HD community has given him a level of maturity he doesn't see in others his age. He is now more open about his own experiences, he's gained new social skills, and he relies on hope. "Hope plays an essential role. If we don't have hope, it's hard to have that drive and passion to do something about this," he said. "If there's no hope, then it's a lot easier to focus on the negative. Being hopeful and positive gives me a chance to make an impact for others and help end this suffering and find the cure. Hope keeps us going."

Making a difference

Would you live life differently if you knew your life would be shortened by a debilitating disease? It's only natural to wonder what you would do if you were in another person's shoes. Perhaps you think you would embrace the possibility of a future in which you might have Huntington's disease and do everything you could to fill the rest of your presymptomatic life with rich experiences – you'd create your bucket list and start checking off the items.

When I was at risk for Huntington's disease, it never occurred to me to make such a list. I didn't decide to travel the world or seek out memorable experiences. There was nothing about the possibility of limited time that inspired me to look for adventure. Instead, I was preoccupied with what the future held for me and my family, so my priorities were learning about Huntington's disease and figuring out how to cope.

Instead of creating a bucket list, I thought a lot about what was important in my life – what gave my life meaning. I focused on spending time with my family, making smart decisions, and making a point of mixing a little fun into my day-to-day responsibilities. Nothing grand. While we all want to live a life full of rich experiences, what we need even more is to connect with each other and live a life that matters. I couldn't change the fact that I belong to an HD family, but I could connect with others and contribute to the greater good. I attended a support group sporadically for a few years and helped launch an annual fundraising walk. These were small things, but important all the same to helping me cope.

Looking ahead to a future affected by Huntington's disease can be paralyzing, or it can motivate you to make purposeful decisions – intentional decisions – about what you want life to look like. Living an intentional life is not easy. It doesn't make up for what's been lost by any means, but when faced with a disease that is debilitating to the entire family, sometimes the only thing you can do is try to find meaning and purpose in how you respond. Lauren Hagenmeyer is a gene-positive young woman from North Carolina who spoke eloquently about how making a difference in others' lives gives her own life value.

Lauren was very young when her mom started having HD symptoms that included substance abuse and abusing Lauren and her siblings. Lauren's parents divorced when she was a baby, and the family moved in with Lauren's grandma when her mom was no longer able to perform the duties of her nursing job. Eventually, Lauren was removed from the home and one of her older siblings became her guardian. Her mom died of Huntington's disease several years ago.

Growing up, Lauren doesn't remember anyone in her family talking about Huntington's disease, not even her grandma. She had no explanation for her mom's symptoms until her older sister eventually told her their mom had Huntington's disease. Lauren didn't talk to anyone outside the family about Huntington's disease until she connected with a support group after she finished college. Now, she finds a lot of support within the HD community, and she finds comfort in being around others who understand. She likes being *boring* when she attends HD conferences. "It's nice to be understood," she said. "It's nice to have the fellowship. It's nice to get involved and be part of something."

Lauren would like to see more public awareness of Huntington's disease. "It can be incredibly isolating, even if you're surrounded by people – especially if you're surrounded by people, to be honest. Most people do not understand," she said. "The best way to destigmatize Huntington's is for there to be more public education. When you destigmatize something, you're more likely to be treated with sympathy and accepted into a community."

Lauren's sense of purpose is a positive part of her life. "I want to be seen and heard as someone in the HD community, and I want to be an advocate on behalf of people with other minority diseases that don't get much attention or have too much stigma," she said. "So that means participating in walks for ALS, for example. You might argue that it's a different disease, so it's not my problem. It's still a heartache; it's still incurable; it's still my brother and sister in humanity. So yes, it is my problem."

When Lauren decided to get tested for Huntington's disease, she went through the process alone because she didn't think her family would support her decision. She was by herself when she received her genetic test result. When Lauren learned she was gene positive, she was more concerned for the genetic counselor than for herself. "I remember feeling sorry for my genetic counselor because he looked so pained," she said. "You'd think that news – that worst-case scenario – would make me cry, but it didn't. The whole thing was strangely undramatic and unpretentious, honestly."

Lauren thinks her depression has eased since learning her gene status. "When you don't know, you are diagnosing and un-diagnosing yourself several times a day," she said. "If you accidentally drop a plate, you must have Huntington's. If you can walk in a straight line and perform all your duties at work, you clearly don't have Huntington's. Eventually, all that back-and-forth makes you sick. So, even though there is no cure, I feel better knowing." While Lauren is glad to know her gene status, she wishes she hadn't shared her positive result with her mom before her mom passed away. "That's one of my big regrets," Lauren said. "I wish I hadn't... but I did."

Soon after receiving her positive test result, and just before the COVID-19 pandemic set in, Lauren left her good friends and small town behind to move to North Carolina. Lauren doesn't drive, so she wanted to live in a city where she could have easy access to a larger community. "For the time being, my legs can still walk and take me where I need to go, and that's important to me," she said. Lauren lives closer to her family now and spends more time with them, especially her sisters' kids. "One of the things that kills me the most, honestly, is knowing that my niece and nephews are going to look at me differently later in life," Lauren said. "I want to give them as many good memories as possible, because it is an ugly trainwreck of a disease."

Lauren's gene-positive status affects her interactions with her family.

She is the youngest of five kids. Two of her sisters are gene negative, one sister is at risk, and her brother has autism and doesn't understand enough about Huntington's disease to get tested. Lauren knows that genetic testing isn't for everyone, but it is hard for her to relate to her sister who is still at risk because Lauren doesn't want to go back to not knowing. She also thinks being gene positive sets her apart from her gene-negative sisters. They know what it's like to be at risk, but they don't know what it's like to be gene positive. "My confirmed-negative siblings and I can't look at each other the same way again," she said. "Our realities are different."

Now that she knows she's gene positive, Lauren thinks a lot about how to approach her life. "I am called to live more urgently and more presently because I know that life is going to be a lot shorter," she said. "I've come to the place where I don't regret the idea of dying young so much as I fear the idea of living a life that I was ashamed to live." One place Lauren finds meaning is participating in research. When we spoke, she was days away from participating in a study that involved getting a lumbar puncture and MRI, along with assessments to measure her fine motor skills, memory, and quality of life. "I think sitting still for an hour is going to be hard, but I want to contribute something," she said.

It is important to Lauren to have a job that makes a difference in others' lives, so she teaches at a daycare. She finds hope in contributing to a better life for others, even if those contributions are small. Thinking about her future, Lauren said, "I'm self-contradictory on the subject. I'm both fatalistic and hopeful. I believe that if I have a meaningful job doing something that matters, that will bring value to my life and existence. I believe it's possible for a cure to be developed in my lifetime, but I also know that as I get older – I'm going to be 29 this year – I don't want to think I can bribe my way out of death. I want to be a good person. I want to do good things. I'm not extraordinary in that respect."

Lauren also talked about hope. "I do look for it. I know that with the time I have left, I can do fundraisers, and I can contribute to Huntington's disease by being in studies. These are arguably small things, and maybe they're even futile things, but you need to believe in something," she said. "I would like to approach the end – however it happens – with a conviction that people are good. It does feel good to live for something. One blessing that comes from being in the Huntington's disease community is if you're going to survive, you are going to have to live with conviction on behalf of something, some cause. No matter how grand or trite it is, it just matters that it exists, and you contribute something to it."

Thinking ahead to her future, Lauren said, "One day, I hope there is a world where Huntington's disease is gone. I don't know if I will live to see it, but I know that while I can still walk to the grocery store and back, I call it a tiny triumph. Even if my work can be exhausting, it does matter. Even if the kids won't remember me because they are too young – even if, in the end, most of my memories are going to spill into the sea of memory – at least they will have existed even once. The best way for me to live is to be hopeful, but not naïve."

Hope and meaning play a significant role in the HD community. It would be hard to get through the most difficult parts of the HD journey without the lifeline they provide. However, it is important to recognize that there are different kinds of hope. When hope lies in something that is beyond our control – like hoping researchers will find a treatment or cure in time – it feels elusive because it's up to others to make those things happen.

But when hope resides in something we can be a part of – like participating in research, spreading awareness, or connecting with others – it is empowering and meaningful. Many *Livable Lives* storytellers are determined to make a difference for their loved ones and others in the HD community. So, too, are the many HD advocates around the world who work tirelessly to support the HD community, change health policy, and push research forward. Even if their efforts may not benefit themselves, they are compelled to help those coming after them. *They create hope through their actions.*

It is also important to recognize that hope can be hard to hold onto in the HD world; it comes and goes, but it's there. It is present in each of the stories shared with me – stories in which people actively create and maintain a livable life in the face of enormous challenges. As I interact with more and more people in the HD community, I am not exaggerating when I say I see the very best of humanity in them. *They give me hope.*

FINAL REFLECTIONS

My mom died shortly after I began my conversations with the HD community. I grieved her loss as I transcribed these stories. I'm grateful I recorded several conversations with her in the year before she died. I love hearing her voice. Even though our conversations were about my family's HD experience, there are moments of laughter that make me happy when I listen to them.

As I sorted items from my mom's bedroom closet the summer after she passed away, I found a small wooden box of letters my dad wrote to her between the time they met and their wedding day six months later. My dad's excitement was over-the-top. He was so happy to have her in his life and often referred to the number of days – the number of hours – until their wedding:

"Only 3 weeks plus one day – yahoooo!"
"I wish I could snap my fingers and have the 360 hours behind us."
"Twelve miserable days, and then I'll be there."

As I read letter after letter, I didn't recognize the person who wrote them. My dad was engaged, optimistic, and gushing about how much he loved my mom. How many ways can you tell someone you cannot wait to get married? It turns out, there are many!

Ever since my mom died, I like to picture my parents greeting each other after decades apart. I imagine that, once again, my dad couldn't wait to be with my mom. She has so much to share with him. She can tell him why his world became so difficult and confusing and why his dad wasn't himself in his later years. She can also tell my dad about each of their grandkids, most of whom he never met. I like to think my dad's mind is clear and sharp, and my mom is reacquainting herself with the life partner she knew and loved when they were young; and they can truly get to know each other once again.

If my dad had not had Huntington's disease and if he hadn't died of cancer, he'd be in his 80s now. He would have been a part of family gatherings and conversations over the years, and he wouldn't be a mystery to me. My kids would have grown up with a grandpa who I think would have been fun, kind, and involved in their lives. I still want to know my dad better and find things we have in common. I wish I could do that by spending time with him, but that opportunity vanished long ago.

I'm starting to understand that connecting with my dad isn't so much about re-creating the father I never knew and imagining the what-ifs of how my family would be different if he hadn't had Huntington's disease. Instead, I can learn a lot by understanding what his life was like and accepting him for who he was, Huntington's disease and all. In the end, my own HD story is much more than a story of loss. My story is an ongoing exploration of what it means to belong to an HD family, and perhaps more importantly, what it means to me to live my livable life. What I know for certain is that there's value in living a good life – one in which we care for and connect with our loved ones and try our best to make a difference.

EPILOGUE: A LIVABLE LIFE

When I first heard Brianna mention the term *livable life*, I knew it was an important concept. She had given a name to an idea that resonates in the HD community: the idea that belonging to an HD family makes you consider what's important in your own life.

When I spoke with Brianna again two years later, I learned that the way she thinks about her own livable life has changed. "The term has definitely evolved in my brain," she said. "Back then? I was still coping with the knowledge that my life will be different than that of my friends. I wanted to use this short period of time to the fullest." And Brianna has done that. "But now," she continued, "even though I know my life will be cut short due to Huntington's, it gives me the opportunity to live a little less encumbered by the what-ifs of tomorrow."

She hopes her *livable life* term will inspire others in the HD community and encourage more conversations. "While living with HD is hard," she said, "it doesn't have to be the death sentence so many people focus on. It's important to find the little things that make each day worth living and make each year mean something. I want people to remember to look for those good moments, even when they're in the thick of Huntington's and things seem the toughest. I think that's what living a *livable life* means to me."

What does a *livable life* mean to you?

Please follow along and share photos
and stories of your own livable life.

#LivableLives
Instagram @christydearien

ENDNOTES

HD 101

GENETICS

NOTE: Global differences in Huntington's disease prevalence may be due to variations in diagnostic criteria and access to care.

CITATIONS:

Huntington's Disease Society of America (HDSA). "What is HD?" Accessed April 2024, https://hdsa.org/what-is-hd/.

Huntington's Disease Youth Organization (HDYO). "What is HD?" Accessed April 2023, https://en.hdyo.org/a/57-what-is-huntington-s-disease.

Mayo Clinic. "Diseases and Conditions: Huntington's Disease." Accessed April 2023, https://www.mayoclinic.org/diseases-conditions/huntingtons-disease/symptoms-causes/syc-20356117.

Myers, R.H. 2004. "Huntington's Disease Genetics." *The Journal of the American Society for Experimental NeuroTherapeutics* 1:255-262. DOI: 10.1602/neurorx.1.2.255.

GENE STATUS

CITATIONS:

Forrest Keenan, K., L. McKee, and Z. Miedzybrodzka. 2014. "Help or Hindrance: Young People's Experiences of Predictive Testing for Huntington's Disease." *Clinical Genetics* 87(6):563-569. DOI: 10.1111/cge.12439.

Jones, Randi. 1996. *Walking the Tightrope: Living At risk for Huntington's Disease.* Huntington's Disease Society of America, New York, NY.

HD SYMPTOMS

CITATIONS:

Bird, Thomas D. 2019. *Can You Help Me? Inside the Turbulent World of Huntington Disease.* Oxford University Press. Kindle.

Harmon, Amy. 2007. "Facing Life with a Lethal Gene." *The New York Times*, March 18, 2007.

Higgs, Laquita M., and Elton D. Higgs. 2019. *Shattered Dreams but Hope: Encouragement for Caregivers of Huntington's Disease and Other Progressive Illnesses.* Elm Hill, Nashville, TN. Kindle.

Huntington's Disease Society of America (HDSA). "Age of Onset." Accessed April 2023, https://hdsa.org/what-is-hd/age-of-onset/.

Huntington's Disease Society of America (HDSA). 2016. *Genetic Testing Protocol for Huntington's Disease.* HDSA, New York.

Huntington's Disease Society of America (HDSA). "Huntington's Disease Symptoms." Accessed April 2023, https://hdsa.org/what-is-hd/huntingtons-disease-symptoms/.

HDYO, "What is HD?"

Kachian, Z.R., S. Cohen-Zimerman, D. Bega, B. Gordon, and J. Grafman. 2019. "Suicidal Ideation and Behavior in Huntington's Disease: Systematic Review and Recommendations." *Journal of Affective Disorders* 250:319-329. DOI: 10.1016/j.jad.2019.03.043.

Li. J., Y. Wang, R. Yang, W. Ma, J. Yan, Y. Li, G. Chen, and J. Pan. 2023. "Pain in Huntington's disease and its potential mechanisms." *Frontiers in Aging Neuroscience* 15:1190563. DOI: 10.3389/fnagi.2023.1190563.

Mayo Clinic, "Diseases and Conditions: HD."

Raven, Charlotte. 2021. *Patient 1: Forgetting and Finding Myself*. Jonathan Cape, London.

Riksförbundet Huntingtons Sjukdom (Swedish Huntington Association). 2023. "Basic Training on Huntington's Disease." Accessed August 2023, https://huntington.se/utbildningar/vara-webbutbildningar/basic-training-english-version/.

Welsh, E., and E. Allmann Updyke. 2021. "Episode 69 – Huntington's Disease: Let's Talk Frankly." *This Podcast will Kill You*. Aired March 23, 2021, http://thispodcastwillkillyou.com/2021/03/23/episode-69-huntingtons-disease-lets-talk-frankly/.

Wheelock, V., L. Scher, B.J. Kocsis, T. Tempkin, and L. Mooney. 2021. *Behavior & Mood Symptoms in HD: Strategies for Patients and Families*. HDSA Center of Excellence at UC Davis Health, Davis, CA.

DISEASE PROGRESSION

CITATIONS:

Burtscher, J., B. Strasser, G. Pepe, M. Burtscher, M. Kopp, A. Di Pardo, V. Maglione, and A.V. Khamoui. 2024. "Brain Periphery Interactions in Huntington's Disease: Mediators and Lifestyle Interventions." *International Journal of Molecular Science* 25(9): 4696. DOI: 10.3390/ijms25094696.

Huntington's Disease Society of America (HDSA). "Huntington's Disease Stages." Accessed April 2023, https://hdsa.org/what-is-hd/huntingtons-disease-stages/.

International Huntington Association. "Huntington's Disease." Accessed April 2023, https://huntington-disease.org/new-to-huntingtons-disease-2/.

A BRIEF HISTORY

NOTES: 1) George Huntington's description of chorea was first published in the *Medical and Surgical Reporter of Philadelphia* on April 13, 1872. 2) Dr. Nancy Wexler revealed in 2020 that she is gene positive. 3) Because of their geographic isolation, the Venezuelan families that made the discovery of the genetic mutation that causes Huntington's disease possible may be unlikely to receive care if effective treatments are ever developed. A nonprofit called Factor H raises funds to support them.

CITATIONS:
Cleveland Clinic. "Should You Get Genetic Testing for Huntington's Disease?" Accessed April 2023, https://health.clevelandclinic.org/genetic-testing-for-huntingtons-disease.
Encyclopedia Britannica. "Eugenics." Accessed April 2023, https://www.britannica.com/science/eugenics-genetics.
Grady, Denise. 2020a. "Haunted by a Gene." *The New York Times*, March 10, 2020.
Grady, Denise. 2020b. "A Second Interview with Dr. Nancy Wexler, 30 Years Later." *The New York Times*, March 10, 2020.
Huntington's Disease Society of America (HDSA). "History of Huntington's Disease." Accessed April 2023, https://hdsa.org/what-is-hd/history-and-genetics-of-huntingtons-disease/history-of-huntingtons-disease/.
Wexler, Alice. 2008. *The Woman Who Walked into the Sea: Huntington's and the Making of a Genetic Disease*. Yale University Press, New Haven & London.

A FAMILY DISEASE

MULTIPLE FAMILY MEMBERS ARE AFFECTED

INTERVIEW: My conversation with Jim took place in February 2022.

A SPOUSE'S PERSPECTIVE

INTERVIEW: My conversation with Zoey took place in February 2022.

CITATIONS:
Decruyenaere, M., G. Evers-Kiebooms, A. Boogaerts, K. Demyttenaere, R. Dom, and J.-P. Fryns. 2005. "Partners of Mutation-carriers for Huntington's Disease: Forgotten Persons?" *European Journal of Human Genetics* 13:1077-1085.

A PARENT'S PERSPECTIVE

INTERVIEW: My conversation with Lindsay took place in February 2022.

NOTE: While HD organizations provide guidance for talking with kids about Huntington's disease, there is little scholarly research on the experience of parenting children who are at risk or gene positive.

A CHILD'S PERSPECTIVE

INTERVIEW: My conversation with Anne Elizabeth Saldarriaga Vélez Magnusson took place in January 2022.

CITATIONS:
Forrest, McKee, and Miedzybrodzka, "Help or Hindrance."
Huntington's Disease Youth Organization (HDYO). 2021. "Being a Young Carer."
    Accessed November 2023, https://en.hdyo.org/a/56-being-a-young-carer-en.pdf.
Kjoelaas, S., K.H. Tilleras, and K.B. Feragen. 2020. "The Ripple Effect: A Qualitative Overview of Challenges When Growing Up in Families Affected by

Huntington's disease." *Journal of Huntington's Disease* 9:129-141. DOI: 10.3233/JHD-190377.

Kjoelaas, S., T.K. Jensen, and K.B. Feragen. 2022. "'I knew it wasn't normal, I just didn't know what to do about it': Adversity and caregiver support when growing up in a family with Huntington's disease." *Psychology & Health* 37:2, 211-229. DOI: 10.1080/08870446.2021.1907387.

CHILDREN WITH HUNTINGTON'S DISEASE

CITATIONS:

Eatough, V., H. Santini, C. Eiser, M.L. Goller, W. Krysa, A. de Nicola, M. Paduanello, M. Petrollini, M. Rakowicz, F. Squitieri, A. Tibben, K.L. Weille, B. Landwehrmeyer, O. Quarrell, and J.A. Smith. 2013. "The Personal Experience of Parenting a Child with Juvenile Huntington's Disease: Perceptions across Europe." *European Journal of Human Genetics* 21:1042-1048.

Huntington's Disease Society of America (HDSA). "Juvenile Onset HD." Accessed July 2023, https://hdsa.org/what-is-hd/history-and-genetics-of-huntingtons-disease/juvenile-onset-hd/.

Huntington's Disease Society of America (HDSA). "The Family Guide Series: Juvenile Huntington's Disease." Accessed July 2023, http://hdsa.org/wp-content/uploads/2015/02/juvenile_guide.pdf.

Huntington's Disease Youth Organization (HDYO). "The Basics of JHD." Accessed July 2023, https://www.hdyo.org/a/52-the-basics-of-jhd.

Huntington's Disease Youth Organization (HDYO). "The Difficulty in Diagnosing Juvenile HD." Accessed July 2023, https://www.hdyo.org/a/520-the-difficulty-in-diagnosing-juvenile-hd.

Huntington Society of Canada. "What is Juvenile Huntington Disease?" Accessed July 2023, https://www.huntingtonsociety.ca/learn-about-hd/what-is-juvenile-huntington-disease/.

Mayo Clinic, "Diseases and Conditions: HD."

Moeller, A.A., M.V. Felker, J.A. Brault, L.C. Duncan, R. Hamid, and M.R. Golomb. 2021. "Patients with Extreme Early Onset Juvenile Huntington's Disease Can Have Delays in Diagnosis: A Case Report and Literature Review." *Child Neurology Open* Vol 8. PMCID: PMC8371413. DOI: 10.1177/2329048X211036137.

Oosterloo, M., A. Touze, L.M. Byrne, J. Achenbach, H. Aksoy, A. Coleman, D. Lammert, M. Nance, P. Nopoulos, R. Reilmann, C. Saft, H. Santini, F. Squitieri, S. Tabrizi, J.-M. Burgunder, and O. Quarrell on behalf of the Pediatric Huntington's Disease Working Group of the European Huntington Disease Network. 2024. "Clinical Review of Juvenile Huntington's Disease." *Journal of Huntington's Disease* 13(2):149-161. DOI: 10.3233/JHD-231523.

Quarrell, O.W.J., M.A. Nance, P. Nopoulos, J.S. Paulsen, J.A. Smith, and F. Squitieri. 2013. "Managing Juvenile Huntington's Disease." *Neurodegenerative Disease Management* 3(3). DOI: 10.2217/nmt.13.18.

Quigley, J. 2016. "Juvenile Huntington Disease: Rare but with Psychiatric Implications." *Psychiatric Times* 33(4).

Rarest of the Rare

INTERVIEW: My conversation with Bill and Karen took place in January 2022.

NOTE: A survey of 301 parents of children with rare diseases found that these parents have similar unmet needs even though their children may have different diseases. Parents were dissatisfied with medical professionals' knowledge of rare diseases (54 percent were dissatisfied with how much medical professionals knew about or understood their child's illness). Parents' finances and ability to work were affected by their child's disease (45 percent struggled financially; 38 percent reduced their work hours to care for their child; 34 percent left their job to care for their child). Parents' social connections were affected by their child's disease (75 percent had no contact with other parents with children with the same disease; 46 percent reported feeling socially isolated and lonely; 42 percent did not have access to a disease-specific support group). For more information, see: Pelentsov, L.J., A.L. Fielder, T.A. Laws, and A.J. Esterman. 2016. "The Supportive Care Needs of Parents with a Child with a Rare Disease: Results of an Online Survey." *BMC Family Practice* 17:88. DOI: 10.1186/s12875-016-0488-x.

CITATIONS:
Eatough et al., "The Personal Experience of Parenting a Child."
HDSA, "Age of Onset."
HDSA, "The Family Guide Series: JHD."
International Huntington's Association. "Juvenile Huntington's Disease (JHD)." Accessed July 2023, https://huntington-disease.org/juvenile-huntingtons-disease-jhd/.
National Institutes of Health, Genetic and Rare Diseases Information Center. "Juvenile Huntington disease." Accessed July 2023, https://rarediseases.info.nih.gov/diseases/10510/juvenile-huntington-disease.
Quarrell et al., "Managing Juvenile Huntington's Disease."
Quarrell, O., K.L. O'Donovan, O. Bandmann, and M. Strong 2012. "The Prevalence of Juvenile Huntington's Disease: A Review of the Literature and Meta-Analysis." *PLoS Curr*. DOI: 10.1371/4f8606b742ef3.
Quigley, "Juvenile Huntington Disease."

Shining Light on a Rare Disease

INTERVIEW: My conversation with Londen Tabor took place in March 2023.

NOTE: Information about ChANGE-HD can be found at https://medicine.uiowa.edu/psychiatry/research/change-hd.

CITATIONS:
Eatough et al., "The Personal Experience of Parenting a Child."
HDSA, "The Family Guide Series: JHD."
HDYO, "The Basics of JHD."
HDYO, "The Difficulty of Diagnosing JHD."

Quigley, "Juvenile Huntington Disease."

RELATING TO A LOVED ONE WITH HUNTINGTON'S DISEASE

CONNECTING WITH AN HD PARENT

INTERVIEW: My first conversation with Finn took place in July 2021. We had a follow-up conversation in April 2023.
CITATIONS:
Huntington's Disease Youth Organization (HDYO). "Living in a Family with HD." Accessed February 2024, https://www.hdyo.org/a/62-living-in-a-family-with-hd.

RELATIONSHIPS CHANGE AS SYMPTOMS PROGRESS

INTERVIEW: My first conversation with Ashley Clarke took place in January 2022. We had a follow-up conversation in January 2023. Her *I'm Not Drunk Lifestyle Blog* can be found at https://www.imnotdrunklifestyleblog.co.uk/.
CITATIONS:
Kjoelaas, Jensen, and Feragen, "I knew it wasn't normal."

TALKING ABOUT HUNTINGTON'S DISEASE

STIGMA STIFLES OPENNESS

INTERVIEW: My conversation with Megha Bhaduri took place in January 2022.
NOTE: In the United States, the Affordable Care Act ensures people cannot be denied health insurance due to a pre-existing condition. See https://www.hhs.gov/healthcare/about-the-aca/pre-existing-conditions/index.html.
CITATIONS:
Quaid, K.A., S.L. Sims, M.M. Swenson, J.M. Harrison, C. Moskowitz, N. Stepanov, G.W. Suter, and B.J. Westphal. 2008. "Living at Risk: Concealing Risk and Preserving Hope in Huntington Disease." *Journal of Genetic Counseling* 17(1):117-128. DOI: 10.1007/s10897-007-9133-0.
Welsh and Updyke, "Episode 69 – Huntington's Disease."

TALKING WITH CHILDREN

INTERVIEW: My conversation with Bailey Pratt took place in February 2022.
CITATIONS:
HD Reach. "Parenting: Talking with Children." Accessed February 2024, https://www.hdreach.org/living-well/parenting/parenting.html.

Huntington's Disease Youth Organization (HDYO). "Potential Outcomes of Not Discussing HD." Accessed February 2024, https://www.hdyo.org/a/59-potential-outcomes-of-not-discussing-hd.
Kjoelaas, Tilleras, and Feragen, "The Ripple Effect."
Quaid et al., "Living at Risk."

Difficult Conversations

INTERVIEW: My first conversation with Mallory took place in November 2021. We had a follow-up conversation via email in June 2023.

CITATIONS:
Jones, *Walking the Tightrope*.
Kjoelaas, Tilleras, and Feragen, "The Ripple Effect."
Kjoelaas, Jensen, and Feragen, "I knew it wasn't normal."
Quaid et al., "Living at Risk."
Tilleras, K.H., S.H. Kjoelaas, E. Dramstad, K.B. Feragen, and C. von der Lippe. 2020. "Psychological Reactions to Predictive Genetic Testing for Huntington's Disease: A Qualitative Study." *Journal of Genetic Counseling* 29:1093-1105. DOI: 10.1002/jgc4.1245.

OUTLOOK ON LIFE

A Livable Life

INTERVIEW: My first conversation with Brianna took place in February 2022. Our second conversation took place in July 2024.

Approaching Each Day

INTERVIEW: My conversation with Darcy Hawkins took place in February 2022. Darcy's blog can be found at https://darcynsmith.wixsite.com/flourish/blog.

Important Life Decisions

INTERVIEW: My conversation with Angela took place in January 2022. We had a follow-up conversation in January 2023.

CITATIONS:
Beatty, Steven. 2018. *In-Between Years: Life after a Positive Huntington's Disease Test*. Self-published. Kindle.
Forrest, McKee, and Miedzybrodzka, "Help or Hindrance."
Huntington's Disease Youth Organization (HDYO). 2022. "Being At-risk." Accessed November 2023, https://www.hdyo.org/a/61-being-at-risk.
Quaid, K.A., M.M. Swenson, S.L. Sims, J.M. Harrison, C. Moskowitz, N. Stepanov, G.W. Suter, and B.J. Westphal. 2010. "What Were You Thinking? Individuals At Risk for Huntington Disease Talk About Having Children." *Journal of Genetic Counseling* 19(6):606-617. DOI: 10.1007/s10897-010-9312-2.
Tilleras et al., "Psychological Reactions to Predictive Genetic Testing."

GENETIC TESTING

GENETIC TESTING BASICS

CITATIONS:

Baig, S.S., M. Strong, E. Rosser, N.V. Taverner, R. Glew, Z. Miedzybrodzka, A. Clarke, D. Craufurd, UK Huntington's Disease Prediction Consortium, and O.W. Quarrell. 2016. "22 Years of Predictive Testing for Huntington's Disease: The Experience of the UK Huntington's Prediction Consortium." *European Journal of Human Genetics* 24:1396-1402. DOI: 10.1038/ejhg.2016.36.

Bird, *Can You Help Me?*

Forrest, McKee, and Miedzybrodzka, "Help or Hindrance."

HDSA, *Genetic Testing Protocol*.

Huntington's Disease Youth Organization (HDYO). 2023. "Having Children." Accessed November 2023, https://www.hdyo.org/a/45-having-children.

Lahiri, Nayana. 2011. "Making Babies: Having a Family, the HD Way." *HD Buzz*, July 2, 2011.

Myers, "Huntington's Disease Genetics."

Quaid et al., "What Were You Thinking?"

Quaid et al., "Living at Risk."

Tilleras et al., "Psychological Reactions to Predictive Genetic Testing."

LIVING AT RISK

INTERVIEW: My conversation with Megan took place in February 2022.

CITATIONS:

Baig et al., "22 Years of Predictive Testing."

Chesire, Amy M. 2014. "Ethics of Genetics Testing – A Social Work Perspective." *Social Work Today* 14(1):20.

Forrest, McKee, and Miedzybrodzka, "Help or Hindrance."

Georgetown University. 2019. "Why Adults at Risk for Huntington's Disease Choose Not to Learn if They Inherited Deadly Gene." Georgetown University News Release. Accessed April 2023, https://gumc.georgetown.edu/news-release/why-adults-at-risk-for-huntingtons-disease-choose-not-to-learn-if-they-inherited-deadly-gene/.

Harmon, "Facing Life with a Lethal Gene."

Quaid et al., "Living at Risk."

Raven, *Patient 1*.

THE GENETIC TESTING DECISION

CITATIONS:

Baig et al., "22 Years of Predictive Testing."

The Genetic Testing Process

INTERVIEW: My conversation with Carly took place in January 2022. Our second conversation took place in January 2024.

CITATIONS:
Chesire, "Ethics of Genetics Testing."
HDSA, *Genetic Testing Protocol*.
Huntington's Disease Youth Organization (HDYO). "Genetic Testing Checklist." Accessed February 2024, https://www.hdyo.org/a/570-genetic-testing-checklist.
Myers, "Huntington's Disease Genetics."

Genetic Testing Aftermath

INTERVIEW: My conversation with Samantha took place in February 2022.

CITATIONS:
Chesire, "Ethics of Genetics Testing."
Forrest, McKee, and Miedzybrodzka, "Help or Hindrance."
Hagberg, A, T.-H. Bui, and E. Winnberg. 2010. "More Appreciation of Life or Regretting the Test? Experiences of Living as a Mutation Carrier of Huntington's Disease." *Journal of Genetic Counseling* 20(1):70-79. DOI: 0.1007/s10897-010-9329-6.
Harmon, "Facing Life with a Lethal Gene."
Lawrence, Susan E. 2011. *Just Move Forward: The Simple Truth About Living with Huntington's Disease*. PublishAmerica. Kindle.
Tibben, A. 2007. "Predictive testing for Huntington's disease." *Brain Research Bulletin* 72(2-3):165-171. DOI: https://doi.org/10.1016/j.brainresbull.2006.10.023.
Tilleras et al., "Psychological Reactions to Predictive Genetic Testing."

PROVIDING CARE

Managing symptoms

INTERVIEWS: My conversation with Abby took place in February 2022, and my conversation with Jerry took place in January 2023.

CITATIONS:
Higgs and Higgs, *Shattered Dreams but Hope*.
Petracca, M., S. Di Tella, M. Solito, P. Zinzi, M.R. Lo Monaco, G. Di Lazzaro, P. Calabresi, M.C. Silveri, A.R. Bentivoglio. 2022. "Clinical and Genetic Characteristics of Late-onset Huntington's Disease in a Large European Cohort." *European Journal of Neurology* 2022 Jul;29(7):1940-1951. DOI: 10.1111/ene.15340.
Pollard, Jimmy. 2008. *Hurry Up and Wait! A Cognitive Care Companion: Huntington's Disease in the Middle and More Advanced Years*. James J. Pollard, Jr.
Raven, *Patient 1*.
Riksförbundet Huntingtons Sjukdom, "Basic Training."

FAMILY CAREGIVERS

INTERVIEW: My conversation with Amy took place in February 2022. Her update comes from an email exchange in November 2023.

NOTE: HDYO's *Huntington's Disease: The Impact on Young People* video can be found at https://www.youtube.com/watch?v=P2A0bGMDZW4.

CITATIONS:
Higgs and Higgs, *Shattered Dreams but Hope*.
HDYO, "Being a Young Carer."
Jones, *Walking the Tightrope*.
Kjoelaas, Tilleras, and Feragen, "The Ripple Effect."

TRANSITIONING TO LONG-TERM CARE

INTERVIEW: My conversation with Melissa took place in July 2023.

CITATIONS:
Bird, *Can You Help Me?*
Crutcher-Marin, Therese. 2017. *Watching Their Dance: Three Sisters, a Genetic Disease and Marrying into a Family at Risk for Huntington's*. NorCal Publishing Company, Kindle.
Higgs and Higgs, *Shattered Dreams but Hope*.
Pollard, *Hurry Up and Wait!*
Riksförbundet Huntingtons Sjukdom, "Basic Training."

QUALITY CARE

INTERVIEW: My conversation with Carina Hvalstedt took place in February 2023.

CITATIONS:
Bird, *Can You Help Me?*
Riksförbundet Huntingtons Sjukdom, "Basic Training."

RESEARCH

CITATIONS:
National Organization for Rare Disorders. "Rare Disease Day." Accessed February 2024, https://rarediseases.org/rare-disease-day/.
National Organization for Rare Disorders. "Rare Disease Cures Accelerator (RDCA-DAP)." Accessed March 2024, https://rarediseases.org/rdca-dap/.

LABORATORY RESEARCH

INTERVIEWS: My first conversation with Dr. Srinageshwar took place in January 2022, and we had a follow-up conversation in January 2023. My conversation with Dr. Rossignol took place in January 2022. My conversation with Dr. Dunbar took place in February 2023. I spoke with all three again in December 2023. Dr. Gary Dunbar is the John G. Kulhavi Endowed Professor and E. Malcolm Field Endowed

Chair of Neuroscience at CMU. For more information on their research, visit https://www.cmich.edu/academics/colleges/college-of-medicine/research/basic/rossignol-lab/rossignol-research.

NOTE: The FDA defines gene therapy as modifying or manipulating the expression of a gene to treat or cure disease. This can be done by replacing or inactivating a disease-causing gene or by introducing a new or modified gene. Scientists are exploring several gene therapy products including plasmid DNA, viral vectors, bacterial vectors, human gene editing technology, and patient-derived cellular gene therapy products. Taken from: U.S. Food & Drug Administration. "What is Gene Therapy?" Accessed November 2023, from https://www.fda.gov/vaccines-blood-biologics/cellular-gene-therapy-products/what-gene-therapy.

CITATIONS:
Chiricozzi, E., G. Lunghi, E. Di Biase, M. Fazzari, S. Sonnino, and L. Mauri. 2020. "GM1 Ganglioside is a Key Factor in Maintaining the Mammalian Neuronal Functions Avoiding Neurodegeneration." *International Journal of Molecular Science* 21(3):868. DOI: 10.3390/ijms21030868.

Huntington's Disease Society of America. "Therapies in Pipeline." Accessed March 2024, https://hdsa.org/hd-research/therapies-in-pipeline/.

Lahue R.S. 2020. "New developments in Huntington's Disease and Other Triplet Repeat Diseases: DNA Repair Turns to the Dark Side." *Neuronal Signal* Nov 16;4(4):NS20200010. DOI: 10.1042/NS20200010.

Niccolini, F., and M. Politis. 2014. "Neuroimaging in Huntington's Disease." *World Journal of Radiology* 28;6(6):301-12. DOI: 10.4329/wjr.v6.i6.301.

Oikemus SR, Pfister EL, Sapp E, Chase KO, Kennington LA, Hudgens E, Miller R, Zhu LJ, Chaudhary A, Mick EO, Sena-Esteves M, Wolfe SA, DiFiglia M, Aronin N, Brodsky MH. 2022. "Allele-Specific Knockdown of Mutant Huntingtin Protein via Editing at Coding Region Single Nucleotide Polymorphism Heterozygosities." *Human Gene Therapy* Jan;33(1-2):25-36. DOI: 10.1089/hum.2020.323.

Pradhan, S., R. Gao, K. Bush, N. Zhang, Y.P. Wairkar, and P.S. Sarkar. 2022. "Polyglutamine Expansion in Huntingtin and Mechanism of DNA Damage Repair Defects in Huntington's Disease." *Frontiers in Cellular Neuroscience* Apr 4;16:837576. DOI: 10.3389/fncel.2022.837576.

RESEARCH THAT INCLUDES HD PATIENTS

INTERVIEW: My conversation with Rob Haselberg took place in September 2022.

NOTE: In the United States, the National Institutes of Health defines a clinical trial as: "A research study in which one or more human subjects are prospectively assigned to one or more interventions (which may include placebo or other control) to evaluate the effects of those interventions on health-related biomedical or behavioral outcomes."

CITATIONS:

Andrew, K.M., and L.M. Fox. 2023. "Supporting Huntington's Disease Families Through the Ups and Downs of Clinical Trials." *Journal of Huntington's Disease* 12(1):71-76. DOI: 10.3233/JHD-230565.

Deichmann, R.D., MD, M. Krousel-Wood, MD, MSPH, and J. Breault, MD. 2016. "Bioethics in Practice: Considerations for Stopping a Clinical Trial Early." *Ochsner Journal* 16(3):197-198. PMC5024796.

Harding, Rachel. 2023. "Roche Phase II GENERATION HD2 Study Underway." *HD Buzz*, February 14, 2023.

HDSA, "Therapies in Pipeline."

Molteni, Megan. 2022. "On the Long Road to Treating Huntington's Genetic Stutter, Scientists Return to Overlooked Clues." *Stat*, November 30, 2022.

Sun. D., W. Gao, H. Hu, and S. Zhou. 2022. "Why 90% of clinical drug development fails and how to improve it?" *Acta Pharmaceutica Sinica B* 12(7):3049-3062. DOI: 10.1016/j.apsb.2022.02.002.

US Food & Drug Administration. "Step 3: Clinical Research." Accessed July 2024, https://www.fda.gov/patients/drug-development-process/step-3-clinical-research#Clinical_Research_Phase_Studies.

INCORPORATING THE PATIENT VOICE

INTERVIEW: My conversation with Jenna took place in February 2022.

NOTE: HD-COPE's industry partners include Wave Life Sciences, Roche, Novartis, uniQure, and CHDI, among others.

CITATIONS:

Andrew and Fox, "Supporting Huntington's Disease Families."

Kwon, D. 2021. "Failure of Genetic Therapies for Huntington's Devastates Community." *Nature* 593:180. DOI: 10.1038/d41586-021-01177-7.

HOPE AND MEANING

KNOWING EACH OTHER

INTERVIEWS: My initial conversation with Ella and Lily took place in February 2022. My second conversation with Ella took place in December 2023.

CONNECTING WITH OTHERS

INTERVIEW: My conversation with Mackenzie Remillard took place in January 2022.

MAKING A DIFFERENCE

INTERVIEW: My conversation with Lauren Hagenmeyer took place in February 2022.

ACKNOWLEDGMENTS

First and foremost, I want to thank everyone who shared their experiences to help me tell a more complete story of what it means to be impacted by Huntington's disease. The storytellers in *Livable Lives* trusted me with the most personal parts of their HD journey, and I hope I did their stories justice. I am eternally grateful for their generosity, kindness, feedback, and support. One of my goals in writing *Livable Lives* was to educate others about Huntington's disease, but I think I learned just as much myself. Thank you.

I needed to write my own story before I could attempt to write about others' experiences, but I was anxious about letting others know how Huntington's disease has affected me and my family. It was difficult to reveal a part of my life that I had held so close for so long. I tentatively shared an early draft of my first chapter with several family members and friends, all of whom provided a safe space. My mom, Jason Dearien, Brenda Waldrop, Natalie Watrous, Sam Watrous, Debbie Gray, Frances Davies, Tenley Burke, Stephanie Manson, Holly, Soren Newman, and Harriet McQuarie read my early draft and encouraged me to keep going. I want to thank them for their ongoing support and for continuing to ask me about "the book" whenever they have a chance.

When I started this project, I thought it would be hard to find people willing to share their stories, but I was so wrong. I want to thank my niece for posting my request to a private HD Facebook group, and I want to thank Jenna Heilman, the executive director of HDYO, for sharing my request with HDYO ambassadors. Within hours of sharing my request, emails started pouring in from around the world. The response was staggering. I also want to thank Jenna for providing feedback and advice along the way and giving me experience being on the other end of an interview.

I've always enjoyed the editing process. Even though it can be intimidating to ask others to critique my writing, I find it fascinating to see my work through others' eyes. My biggest thank you goes to Brianna Esker and Debbie Gray for their discerning editorial guidance. They asked hard questions, encouraged me to open up even more than I thought I could, and made sure I paid attention to things like timeline and word choice. This book is 10 times better than it could have been because of their willingness to give honest and supportive feedback.

I wanted *Livable Lives* to be relevant to multiple audiences, so I asked several people to provide feedback on the first full draft. They represented members of the HD community – including those who are at risk, gene positive, gene negative, and HD family members – as well as friends not impacted by Huntington's disease: Frances Davies, Brianna Esker, Debbie Gray, Greg Laprade, Seth Rotberg, Bryan Thomson, Brenda Waldrop, Natalie Watrous, and Sam Watrous. I can't thank them enough for investing a significant amount of their time to read *Livable Lives* and tell me where I could make improvements. It was incredibly helpful to see this early version of *Livable Lives* from their perspectives. I also want to thank Wes Solem from HD genetics for reviewing my descriptions of HD inheritance and genetics for clarity and accuracy.

Several people played a significant role in helping me promote this book. I want to thank Maggie Dawkins for creating a remarkable illustration for the book's front cover. She began by asking what I wanted to convey with *Livable Lives* and then created an image that captured my vision so well. Her design laid the groundwork for the public-facing presentation of the book. I want to thank Natalie Quek for creating my website, developing a look-and-feel for social media, designing the book's cover and interior style guide, designing a media kit, and offering advice for promoting the book. Her work is always impeccable, and she is a joy to work with. In addition, I want to thank Ashley Clarke for showing me how to use Canva, Arian May from HelpCureHD for giving me my first in-person opportunity to tell the HD community about *Livable Lives*, Erin Paterson for sharing publishing resources and advice, and Lauren Holder for making my first-ever interview for *Help4HD Live!* as painless as possible.

And finally, I want to thank the people who have played the most important roles in helping me along the way. I want to thank my husband, Jason, for encouraging me to step beyond my comfort zone and for wholeheartedly believing in my ability to tell this story long before I believed it myself. I want to posthumously thank my mom for showing me how to get through the hardest times with strength and grace. I also want to thank my older brother for allowing me to share his story and for caring about how I was affected when I was at risk, even though he was the one facing Huntington's disease head-on. I will do my best to continue sharing our story.

ABOUT THE AUTHOR

Christy lives in Moscow, Idaho, with her husband. Before striking out on her own, she worked for two decades as a research associate at the University of Idaho, where she honed her research, writing, and editing skills. In her free time, she likes to enjoy the outdoors, explore new places, and spend time with friends and family.

Made in the USA
Columbia, SC
07 December 2024